SLEEP APNEA, INSOMNIA & OTHER SLEEP DISORDERS

A Doctor's Practical Guide to Better Sleep & Better Health

Dr Prabhat Das

MD, PhD, FACP

Better Health with Dr Das Series

Hardcover ISBN: 978-1-971672-49-6

Paperback ISBN: 978-1-971672-48-9

eBook ISBN: 978-1-971672-47-2

Printed in the United States of America

Disclaimer

This book is intended solely for educational and informational purposes. It is not meant to replace personal medical advice, diagnosis, or treatment.

Although I am a licensed physician, reading this book does not establish a doctor-patient relationship. Each individual's health condition, medical history, and risk factors are unique. Any medical decision should be made in partnership with your own healthcare professional who understands your specific situation.

Medical science is continually advancing. New research and updated guidelines may lead to changes in recommendations over time.

About the Author

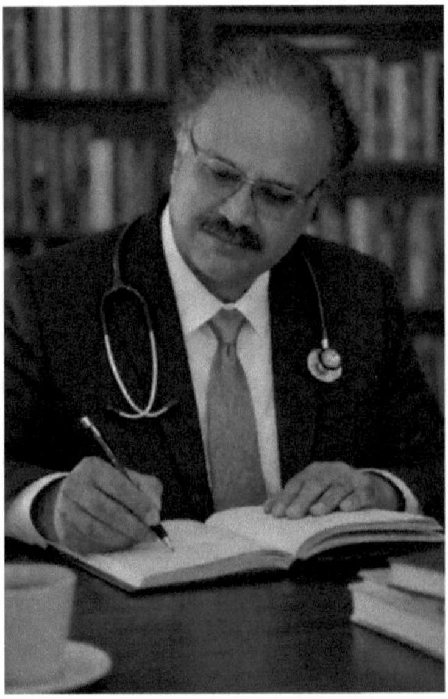

I am Dr Prabhat Das, MD, PhD, FACP. My journey in medicine began in India and, over the past thirty-five years, has continued in the United States, where I have had the privilege of caring for patients across a wide range of medical settings. I am trained in Internal Medicine, Pulmonary Diseases, and Critical Care. For me, medicine has never been just a profession. It has been a lifelong commitment shaped by learning, service, and a deep respect for the trust patients place in their physician.

Over the years, I have had the honor of caring for patients in many different situations. I have seen individuals in my office for routine concerns, treated urgent conditions in busy emergency rooms, managed serious illnesses in the hospital, and cared for critically ill patients in intensive care units. Each setting has taught me something valuable. Each patient has added to my understanding of what it truly means to care for another human being.

But one lesson has stood above all others. Medicine is not only about tests, diagnoses, or treatments. It is about people. It is about listening carefully, understanding fears that are often left unspoken, and guiding patients through uncertainty with clarity and compassion. Again and again, I have seen that what people want most is simple, trustworthy information. They want to understand what is happening in their bodies. They want to feel confident about the decisions they are making for their health and for their families.

These experiences have deeply shaped how I think about health, illness, prevention, and the human side of healing.

That is the reason behind the '**Better Health with Dr Das Series'**. Through these books, I hope to reach individuals I may never meet in person but who are searching for clear and reliable guidance. In today's world, health information is everywhere, yet much of it is confusing, overwhelming, and sometimes misleading. My goal is to cut through that noise and present important medical topics in a way that is simple, practical, and reassuring.

Every page of this series is guided by two foundations: reliable scientific knowledge and decades of real-world clinical experience. I want you, the reader, to feel informed, confident, and empowered. Not overwhelmed. Not confused. But clear about what you can do, step by step, to improve your health.

If even one reader feels less anxious, more informed, or better prepared to take control of their health after reading these books, then this work has served its purpose.

Helping people live healthier, longer, more confident and better-informed lives remains one of the greatest privileges of my life.

Table of Contents:

CHAPTER 1: Why Good Sleep Is One of the Most Powerful Medicines

Sleep Is Not Rest. It Is Repair

In my years of medical practice, I have noticed something very consistent.

Patients become very serious about their health when they are diagnosed with a condition. They begin to monitor their blood pressure, control their sugar, improve their diet, and start exercising. All of this is good and necessary.

But one essential pillar of health is still often ignored.

That pillar is sleep.

Most people think of sleep as a passive activity. They feel that nothing important happens during sleep. In reality, sleep is one of the most active and essential processes in the body.

While you are sleeping, your body is working quietly and continuously. The brain is organizing memories. Hormones are being regulated. Cells are being repaired. The immune system is strengthening itself.

That is why I often tell my patients a simple truth.

Sleep is not wasted time. It is healing time.

What Happens Inside the Body During Sleep

When you fall asleep, your body does not shut down. It shifts into a different and highly organized mode.

Your brain begins to process everything you experienced during the day. Important information is stored. Unnecessary details are filtered out. Emotional experiences are settled.

At the same time, your body begins repair work. Muscles recover. Tissues heal. Hormones that control growth, appetite, and metabolism are adjusted.

Blood pressure naturally falls during healthy sleep. The heart gets a period of rest. The immune system performs important protective functions.

This is why good sleep leaves you feeling refreshed. It is not just rest. It is restoration.

Doctor's Pearl

Good sleep is like a silent medicine.
You do not feel it working, but you clearly feel the difference when it is missing.

Why Poor Sleep Affects You So Quickly

Most patients first notice the effects of poor sleep the next day.

They wake up feeling heavy. The mind feels slow. Concentration becomes difficult. Even simple tasks require more effort.

Mood changes are common. Irritability increases. Patience decreases. Small problems feel bigger than they are.

Many patients come to me saying, "Doctor, I feel tired all the time," or "I cannot focus like before."

Very often, the problem is not in the brain or the body. It is in the quality of sleep.

The Hidden Long-Term Damage

While the short-term effects are noticeable, the long-term effects are more serious.

Chronic poor sleep can gradually affect almost every system in the body.

It can contribute to:

- High blood pressure
- Diabetes
- Weight gain

- Heart disease
- Depression
- Reduced immunity

Sleep problems are not just nighttime issues. They are whole-body issues.

This is especially important in adults over 40, where sleep often interacts with other health conditions.

Why So Many People Ignore Sleep

One of the biggest problems is that poor sleep develops slowly.

People adjust to it. They begin to accept fatigue as normal.

They say:

- "I have always been a light sleeper"
- "This is just part of aging"
- "Everyone is tired these days"

But these are often misconceptions.

Another reason is modern lifestyle. Late-night screen use, stress, irregular schedules, and constant mental activity all interfere with sleep.

Many people simply do not realize that their daily symptoms are connected to poor sleep.

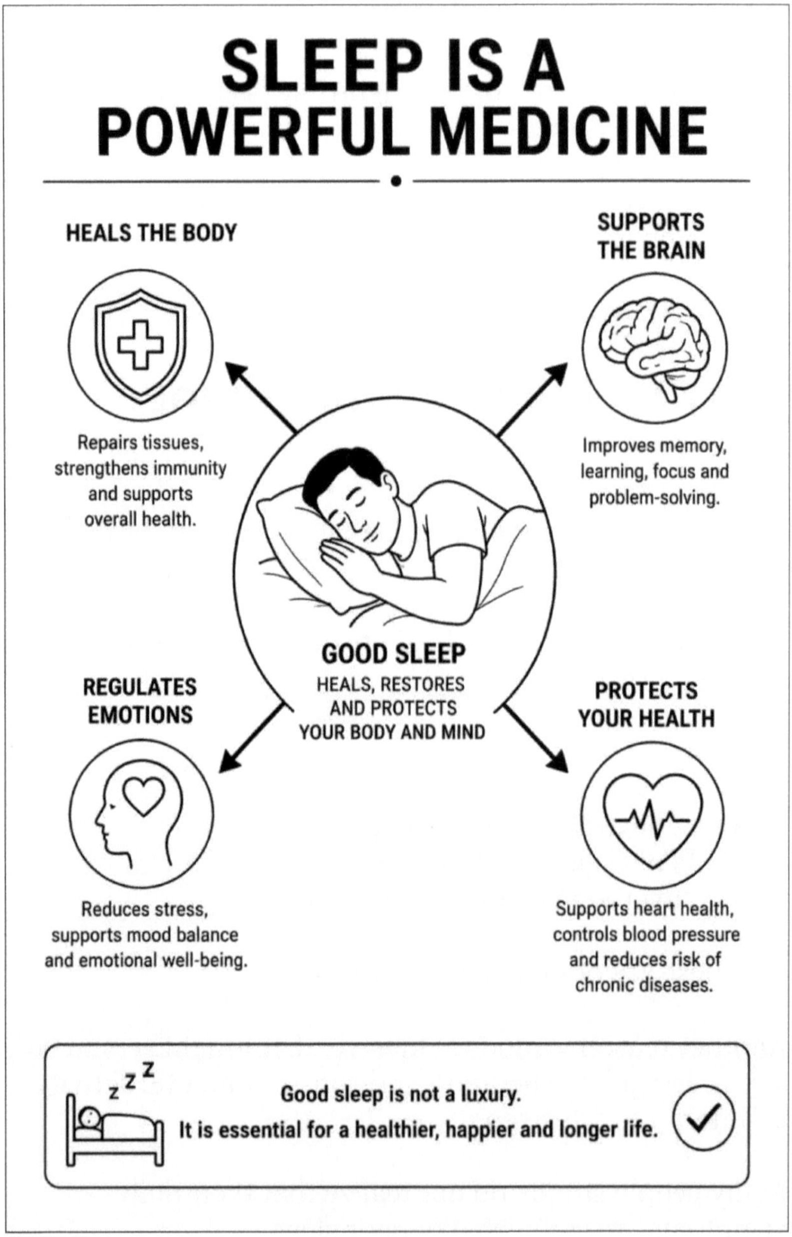
SLEEP IS A POWERFUL MEDICINE
HEALS THE BODY
Repairs tissues, strengthens immunity and supports overall health.
SUPPORTS THE BRAIN
Improves memory, learning, focus and problem-solving.
GOOD SLEEP
HEALS, RESTORES AND PROTECTS YOUR BODY AND MIND
REGULATES EMOTIONS
Reduces stress, supports mood balance and emotional well-being.
PROTECTS YOUR HEALTH
Supports heart health, controls blood pressure and reduces risk of chronic diseases.
z z Z
Good sleep is not a luxury.
It is essential for a healthier, happier and longer life.

Doctor's Pearl

If you wake up tired most days, your body is trying to tell you something.
Do not ignore that message.

What This Book Will Help You Do

This book is written to give you clear, practical understanding.

You will learn:

- What healthy sleep really means
- What can go wrong
- How to recognize sleep disorders
- How sleep affects your overall health
- What practical steps you can take

My goal is simple.

I want you to understand your sleep better and improve it in a way that is realistic and sustainable.

Because when sleep improves, life improves.

Chapter Summary

Sleep is not a passive activity. It is a critical process of repair and restoration.

Poor sleep affects both daily function and long-term health.

Many people ignore sleep problems because they develop gradually.

Sleep should be treated as an essential pillar of health.

Action Plan

- Begin paying attention to your sleep
- Notice how you feel in the morning and during the day
- Identify one habit that may be affecting your sleep
- Do not accept persistent fatigue as normal
- Start treating sleep as a priority

Transition to Chapter 2

Now that you understand why sleep is so important, the next step is to understand how normal sleep actually works.

In the next chapter, we will explore the structure of sleep and what truly healthy sleep looks like.

CHAPTER 2: What Healthy Sleep Really Means

Sleep Is a Structured Process, Not a Passive State

Most people think of sleep as a simple, continuous state. You lie down, fall asleep, and remain asleep until morning.

In reality, sleep is much more organized and dynamic.

During the night, your brain and body move through a series of repeating cycles. Each cycle has different stages, and each stage serves a specific purpose.

This is the reason why two people may both sleep for seven hours, yet one wakes up refreshed and the other feels tired.

It is not only the number of hours that matters. It is how well your sleep is structured.

Understanding the Stages of Sleep

Sleep is broadly divided into two main types:

- Non-REM sleep
- REM sleep

Non-REM sleep has lighter and deeper stages.

In the lighter stages, the body begins to relax. Breathing slows, and the mind starts to drift away from wakefulness.

As sleep deepens, the body enters deep sleep. This is the most physically restorative phase. Muscles relax completely, heart rate slows, and the body focuses on repair.

REM sleep is different. This is the stage where most dreaming occurs. The brain becomes active, almost similar to wakefulness, while the body remains relaxed.

A normal night includes several cycles of these stages, each lasting about 90 minutes.

Deep Sleep and REM Sleep – Both Are Essential

Each stage of sleep plays a unique role.

Deep sleep is mainly for the body. It helps with physical recovery, tissue repair, and immune function.

REM sleep is mainly for the brain. It helps process emotions, improve memory, and sharpen thinking.

If deep sleep is reduced, you may feel physically tired.
If REM sleep is disturbed, you may feel mentally foggy or emotionally unsettled.

Good sleep is not just long sleep. It is balanced sleep.

Doctor's Pearl

If you wake up feeling tired after enough hours of sleep, the problem is often not quantity.
It is the quality of sleep.

The Body Clock – Your Internal Timing System

Your sleep is guided by a natural internal clock called the circadian rhythm.

This clock controls when you feel alert and when you feel sleepy.

It is strongly influenced by light.

Morning light signals the brain to stay awake and active. As evening approaches and light decreases, the body releases melatonin, which prepares you for sleep.

When this rhythm is disrupted, sleep becomes irregular.

Common causes include:

- Late-night screen use
- Irregular sleep schedules
- Shift work
- Frequent travel across time zones

When the body clock is disturbed, even a long sleep may not feel refreshing.

How Much Sleep Do You Really Need?

This is one of the most common questions.

For most adults, the ideal range is about seven to eight hours per night.

However, this is not exact for everyone.

The better way to judge your sleep is by how you feel during the day.

If you are alert, focused, and able to function without excessive fatigue, your sleep is likely adequate.

If you depend on caffeine to stay awake or feel tired most of the day, your sleep may not be sufficient or may not be of good quality.

Doctor's Pearl

Do not count hours alone.
Let your daytime energy tell you whether your sleep is enough.

How Sleep Changes With Age

As people grow older, sleep patterns naturally change.

Sleep may become lighter. There may be more awakenings. It may take longer to fall asleep.

Many older adults also go to bed earlier and wake up earlier.

These changes are common, but they should not be misunderstood.

Poor sleep is not a normal part of aging.

If sleep is consistently disturbed or daytime function is affected, it needs attention.

What Good Sleep Feels Like

It is important to know what healthy sleep actually feels like.

You should:

- Fall asleep within a reasonable time
- Sleep without frequent or prolonged awakenings
- Wake up feeling reasonably refreshed
- Stay alert and functional during the day

Occasional bad nights are normal. What matters is the overall pattern.

Doctor's Pearl

Good sleep is not perfect every night.
It is consistently good over time.

Chapter Summary

Sleep is a structured process with multiple stages that repeat through the night.

Deep sleep restores the body, while REM sleep supports the brain.

The circadian rhythm regulates sleep and wakefulness.

Most adults need about seven to eight hours of sleep, but quality is equally important.

Sleep patterns change with age, but poor sleep is not normal.

Healthy sleep leads to better daytime function.

Action Plan

- Maintain a consistent sleep and wake schedule
- Get natural light exposure in the morning
- Reduce screen exposure in the evening

- Focus on how you feel during the day, not just hours slept
- Avoid irregular sleep patterns

Transition to Chapter 3

Now that you understand what healthy sleep looks like, the next step is to recognize when sleep begins to go wrong.

In the next chapter, we will discuss how sleep problems develop and the early warning signs you should not ignore.

CHAPTER 3: When Sleep Becomes a Problem

A Bad Night Versus a Sleep Disorder

Everyone has a bad night once in a while.

You may have difficulty sleeping because of stress, travel, illness, or a change in routine. The next day may feel slow, but sleep usually returns to normal.

A sleep disorder is different.

It is not occasional. It becomes a pattern. Night after night, sleep is not restful. Day after day, the body begins to feel the effect.

In simple terms, a sleep disorder is present when poor sleep starts affecting how you feel, think, and function during the day.

That is the point where sleep deserves attention.

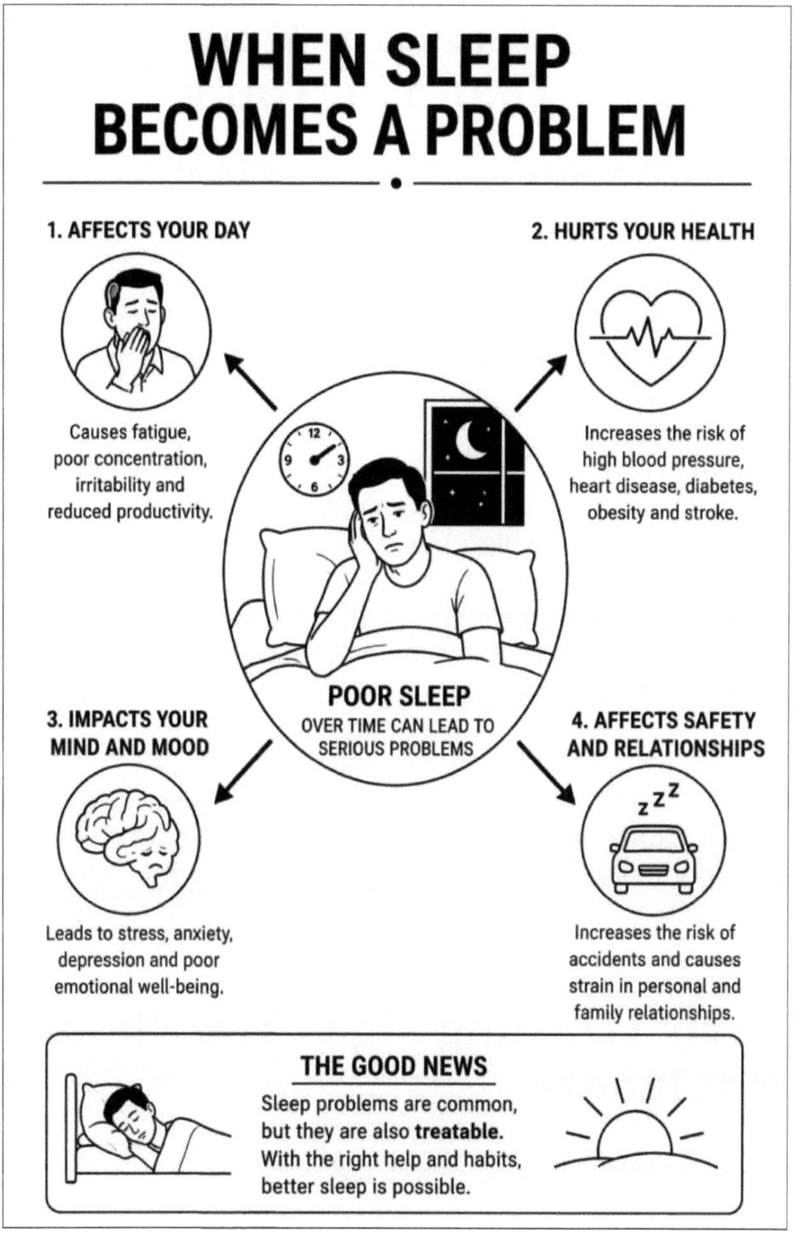
WHEN SLEEP
BECOMES A PROBLEM
1. AFFECTS YOUR DAY
Causes fatigue, poor concentration, irritability and reduced productivity.
2. HURTS YOUR HEALTH
Increases the risk of high blood pressure, heart disease, diabetes, obesity and stroke.
12
9
3
6
POOR SLEEP
OVER TIME CAN LEAD TO SERIOUS PROBLEMS
3. IMPACTS YOUR MIND AND MOOD
Leads to stress, anxiety, depression and poor emotional well-being.
4. AFFECTS SAFETY AND RELATIONSHIPS
z z z
Increases the risk of accidents and causes strain in personal and family relationships.
THE GOOD NEWS
Sleep problems are common, but they are also **treatable.** With the right help and habits, better sleep is possible.

Sleep Problems Are More Common Than You Think

In everyday medical practice, sleep complaints are extremely common.

Some patients come with clear symptoms such as snoring or insomnia. Others come with fatigue, low energy, or poor concentration, without realizing that sleep may be the underlying issue.

Insomnia affects a large number of adults. Sleep apnea is also very common, especially in people who are overweight or have high blood pressure.

Conditions like restless legs syndrome or excessive daytime sleepiness are often overlooked and go undiagnosed for years.

The important thing to understand is this.

You are not alone if you have a sleep problem. But that does not mean it should be ignored.

Early Warning Signs You Should Not Ignore

Sleep problems usually begin quietly.

You may notice that it takes longer to fall asleep. You may start waking up during the night. Sleep may feel lighter than before.

Many people begin to wake up earlier than expected and cannot go back to sleep.

The more important signs often appear during the day.

You may feel tired despite spending enough time in bed. Concentration becomes difficult. Memory may feel less sharp. Irritability increases.

Sometimes, the first sign comes from a partner who notices loud snoring, pauses in breathing, or restless movements.

These early signs are easy to overlook, but they are important.

Doctor's Pearl

If your sleep is affecting your daytime life, it is no longer a minor issue.
It deserves proper attention.

Why People Live With Sleep Problems for Years

One of the most surprising things about sleep disorders is how long people tolerate them.

Many patients gradually adjust their lives around poor sleep. They depend on caffeine. They reduce activity. They accept fatigue as normal.

There is also a tendency to normalize the problem.

People say:

- "This is just how I sleep"
- "It is part of getting older"
- "I am just tired because of work"

These assumptions often delay proper evaluation.

Busy lifestyles add to the problem. Sleep becomes the lowest priority.

Lack of awareness also plays a role. Many people do not connect symptoms like fatigue or irritability with poor sleep.

How Poor Sleep Affects Daily Life

When sleep is disturbed regularly, it begins to affect every part of life.

Work performance declines. Tasks take longer. Mistakes increase.

Mental clarity reduces. Decision-making becomes slower and less accurate.

Mood changes are common. Irritability, anxiety, and emotional sensitivity increase.

Physical energy decreases. Activities that once felt easy become tiring.

There is also an increased risk of accidents, especially while driving.

Poor sleep does not stay confined to the night. It follows you through the day.

Doctor's Pearl

Poor sleep does not just make you tired.
It quietly reduces your ability to perform, think, and respond.

When Should You Seek Medical Help?

A common and important question is when to seek help.

A simple guideline is this.

If a sleep problem lasts more than a few weeks, it should not be ignored.

If you wake up feeling unrefreshed, feel sleepy during the day, or struggle to concentrate, it is time to discuss it with your doctor.

Certain symptoms need earlier attention:

- Loud snoring
- Choking or gasping during sleep
- Observed pauses in breathing
- Sudden daytime sleep episodes
- Unusual behaviors during sleep

Early evaluation makes treatment easier and more effective.

Chapter Summary

A sleep disorder is not an occasional bad night, but a persistent pattern.

Sleep problems are very common but often ignored.

Early warning signs include difficulty falling asleep, frequent awakenings, and daytime fatigue.

Many people live with sleep problems for years due to normalization and lack of awareness.

Poor sleep affects work, mood, safety, and overall health.

Medical evaluation is important when symptoms persist.

Action Plan

- Observe your sleep pattern over the next one to two weeks
- Note any difficulty falling asleep or staying asleep

- Pay attention to your daytime energy and focus
- Ask your partner about snoring or unusual sleep behavior
- Do not ignore symptoms that persist
- Seek medical advice when needed

Transition to Chapter 4

Now that you understand how sleep problems begin and how to recognize them, we will look at the most common sleep disorder in detail.

In the next chapter, we will explore insomnia, why it happens, and how it can be effectively managed.

CHAPTER 4: Insomnia – Why So Many People Struggle to Sleep

Understanding What Insomnia Really Means

In everyday conversation, people often say, "I have insomnia" after a bad night.

But true insomnia is more than an occasional sleepless night.

Insomnia is a persistent difficulty with falling asleep, staying asleep, or waking too early and not being able to return to sleep. Most importantly, it affects how you feel during the day.

Many patients describe it very clearly.

"Doctor, I am in bed for hours, but I cannot sleep."
"I wake up multiple times and never feel rested."
"I wake up early and my sleep is finished for the night."

What matters is not just time spent in bed, but how restful that sleep is.

Different Patterns of Insomnia

Insomnia does not appear the same in everyone.

Some people mainly struggle to fall asleep. They lie awake for long periods, often with an active mind.

Others fall asleep easily but wake up repeatedly during the night. Their sleep becomes fragmented.

Some wake up very early in the morning and cannot return to sleep, even though they still feel tired.

Many patients have a combination of these patterns.

Understanding your pattern is important because it helps guide the right approach to treatment.

Why Insomnia Develops

Insomnia rarely has a single cause. It usually develops from a combination of factors.

Stress is one of the most common triggers. Work pressure, family concerns, and health issues can keep the mind active at night.

Anxiety and depression often contribute. The mind becomes alert when it should be slowing down.

Physical conditions such as chronic pain, acid reflux, breathing problems, or frequent urination can disturb sleep.

Lifestyle habits also play a major role:

- Irregular sleep schedules
- Late-night screen use
- Caffeine intake
- Alcohol use
- Lack of physical activity

With increasing age, sleep becomes lighter, making it easier for these factors to disturb it.

The Vicious Cycle of Insomnia

One of the most important things to understand is how insomnia becomes a cycle.

It often starts with a few poor nights.

Naturally, the person begins to worry about sleep. That worry creates tension at bedtime.

They try harder to sleep. But sleep cannot be forced.

The bed slowly becomes associated with frustration instead of rest.

Many patients say, "The moment I lie down, I become more awake."

This is not because their body cannot sleep. It is because their mind has learned the wrong association.

Breaking this cycle is the key to recovery.

Doctor's Pearl

The more you try to force sleep, the more it moves away from you.
Sleep comes when you allow it, not when you chase it.

How Insomnia Affects Health Over Time

In the beginning, insomnia may feel like an inconvenience.

Over time, it begins to affect many areas of life.

Energy decreases. Concentration becomes difficult. Work performance suffers.

Mood is affected. Irritability, anxiety, and low motivation become more common.

Long-standing insomnia can also contribute to high blood pressure, heart disease, and metabolic problems.

Some patients begin to depend on sleep medications without proper guidance, which can create additional challenges.

Insomnia should not be ignored.

A Healthier Way to Think About Sleep

One of the most helpful shifts I encourage is this.

Do not try to force sleep. Instead, support sleep.

Sleep is not like a switch that you turn on. It is more like a natural process that happens when the body and mind are ready.

When you remove pressure and create the right conditions, sleep begins to return.

This shift alone often brings relief to patients.

Doctor's Pearl

Sleep is not under your control, but your habits are. Change the habits, and sleep begins to change.

Chapter Summary

Insomnia is a persistent difficulty with sleep that affects daytime functioning.

It can appear as difficulty falling asleep, staying asleep, or waking too early.

It usually develops due to a combination of stress, medical conditions, and lifestyle habits.

Insomnia often becomes a self-perpetuating cycle driven by anxiety and learned patterns.

Over time, it affects both mental and physical health.

Improvement begins by changing how we approach sleep.

Action Plan

- Maintain a regular sleep and wake schedule
- Avoid trying to force sleep
- Limit screen exposure before bedtime
- Reduce caffeine, especially later in the day
- Create a calm pre-sleep routine
- Seek help if insomnia persists

Transition to Chapter 5

Insomnia is a condition where sleep is not sufficient or not restful.

However, there are situations where people sleep for many hours but still feel tired because their breathing is repeatedly disturbed during the night.

In the next chapter, we will explore sleep apnea, one of the most common and often undiagnosed sleep disorders.

CHAPTER 5: Sleep Apnea – The Silent Disorder That Drains Your Energy

When You Sleep But Still Feel Exhausted

Many patients come to me with a very similar complaint.

"Doctor, I sleep for seven or eight hours, but I still wake up tired."

At first, this can be confusing. If the duration of sleep is adequate, why does the body still feel exhausted?

In many such cases, the problem is not how long you sleep, but what happens during your sleep.

Sleep apnea is one of the most common reasons for this pattern.

What Sleep Apnea Really Is

Sleep apnea is a condition in which breathing repeatedly becomes interrupted during sleep.

These interruptions may last for several seconds and can occur many times each hour.

The most common type is **obstructive sleep apnea**.

In this condition, the airway becomes narrow or temporarily collapses during sleep. As a result, airflow is reduced or completely blocked for a short period.

The body reacts quickly. It briefly wakes up just enough to reopen the airway.

Most people do not remember these awakenings, but they happen repeatedly through the night.

This breaks the natural sleep cycle and prevents deep, restorative sleep.

Why the Airway Closes During Sleep

When you are awake, the muscles of the throat help keep the airway open.

During sleep, these muscles relax. In some people, this relaxation leads to narrowing or collapse of the airway.

Several factors increase the risk:

- Excess weight, especially around the neck
- A naturally narrow airway
- Enlarged tonsils
- Alcohol or sedative use
- Sleeping on the back
- Increasing age

These factors make it easier for the airway to close during sleep.

Doctor's Pearl

Sleep apnea is not just about snoring.
It is about repeated stress on your body throughout the night.

Who Is at Risk?

Sleep apnea can affect anyone, but certain groups are at higher risk.

Men are more commonly affected, although women are also at risk, especially after menopause.

People who are overweight or obese have a higher chance of developing sleep apnea.

Those with high blood pressure, diabetes, or heart disease should be particularly alert.

Loud, regular snoring is an important clue.

However, I have seen patients who do not fit the typical profile but still have significant sleep apnea. So it should not be ruled out based on appearance alone.

SIGNS & SYMPTOMS OF SLEEP APNEA

Sleep apnea is a condition where breathing repeatedly stops and starts during sleep. Watch for these common signs.

1. LOUD SNORING

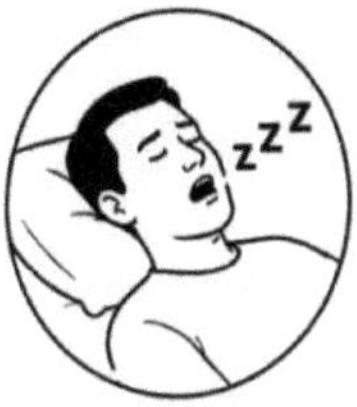

Loud, frequent snoring is the most common sign.

2. PAUSES IN BREATHING

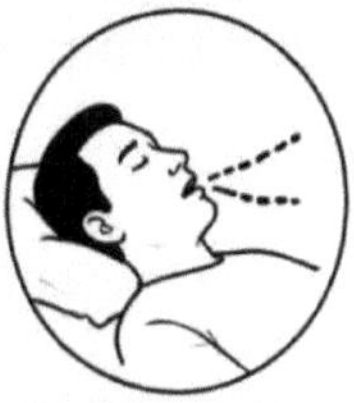

Breathing repeatedly stops for a few seconds and then starts again.

3. GASPING OR CHOKING

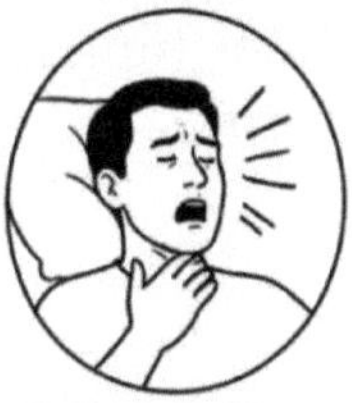

Waking up suddenly gasping or choking during the night.

4. EXCESSIVE DAYTIME SLEEPINESS

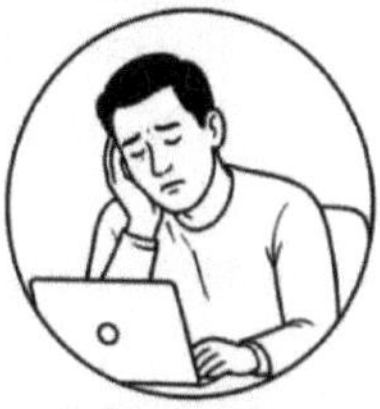

Feeling very sleepy during the day, even after a full night's sleep.

5. MORNING HEADACHE

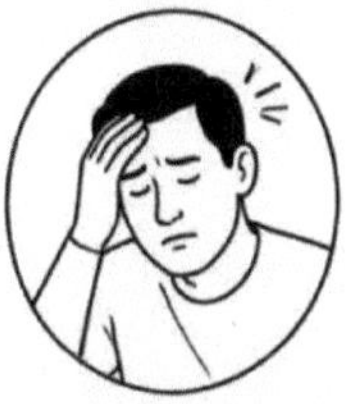

Waking up with headache or a heavy feeling.

6. UNREFRESHED SLEEP

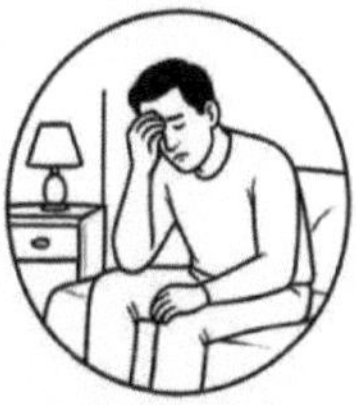

Waking up tired and not feeling refreshed.

7. DIFFICULTY CONCENTRATING

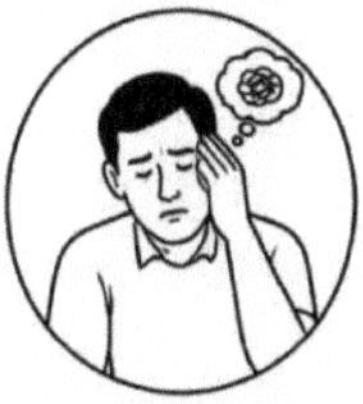

Trouble focusing, forgetfulness and poor concentration.

8. MOOD CHANGES AND IRRITABILITY

Feeling irritable, moody, anxious or depressed.

If you or your bed partner notice these signs, it is important to get evaluated by a doctor.

Early diagnosis and treatment can improve your health and quality of life.

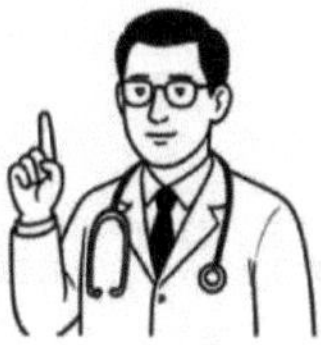

Recognizing the Symptoms

Sleep apnea often shows itself through a combination of night and daytime symptoms.

At night:

- Loud snoring
- Choking or gasping
- Pauses in breathing noticed by a partner
- Restless sleep

In the morning:

- Dry mouth
- Headache
- Feeling unrefreshed

During the day:

- Excessive sleepiness
- Poor concentration
- Irritability
- Low energy

Many patients do not realize these symptoms are connected.

Why Sleep Apnea Often Goes Undiagnosed

One of the challenges with sleep apnea is that it occurs during sleep.

The patient may not be aware of the breathing pauses or repeated awakenings.

Often, it is a spouse or family member who first notices the problem.

Another issue is normalization.

People think snoring is harmless. They blame fatigue on stress or age.

As a result, many patients live with sleep apnea for years without diagnosis.

Doctor's Pearl

If someone tells you that you snore loudly or stop breathing during sleep, take it seriously.
It is not just a noise. It is a warning.

Why Sleep Apnea Is Dangerous

Sleep apnea is not just a sleep disorder. It is a whole-body condition.

Each time breathing stops:

- Oxygen levels drop
- Heart rate increases
- Blood pressure rises

This repeated stress affects the cardiovascular system.

Untreated sleep apnea is linked to:

- High blood pressure
- Heart disease
- Stroke
- Irregular heart rhythms
- Diabetes
- Weight gain

It also affects the brain, leading to poor concentration and increased risk of accidents.

The Good News – It Is Treatable

One of the most encouraging aspects of sleep apnea is that it can be effectively treated.

When properly managed, many patients experience dramatic improvement.

They begin to wake up refreshed. Daytime energy improves. Mental clarity returns.

Some patients even see improvements in blood pressure and overall health.

The key is recognizing the condition and taking the first step toward evaluation.

Chapter Summary

Sleep apnea is a condition where breathing repeatedly stops or becomes shallow during sleep.

Obstructive sleep apnea is caused by airway collapse during sleep.

Risk factors include obesity, age, and anatomical factors, but it can occur in anyone.

Symptoms include snoring, breathing pauses, and daytime fatigue.

It often goes undiagnosed because the patient is unaware of nighttime events.

Untreated sleep apnea has serious health consequences but is highly treatable.

Action Plan

- Do not ignore loud or persistent snoring
- Ask your partner about breathing pauses during sleep
- Pay attention to daytime sleepiness
- Avoid alcohol close to bedtime
- Try sleeping on your side
- Seek medical evaluation if symptoms are present

Transition to Chapter 6

Obstructive sleep apnea is the most common breathing-related sleep disorder.

However, it is not the only one.

In the next chapter, we will explore other breathing-related sleep disorders, including central sleep apnea, and understand how they differ and why accurate diagnosis is important.

CHAPTER 6: Other Breathing Problems During Sleep

When the Problem Is Not a Blocked Airway

In the previous chapter, we discussed obstructive sleep apnea, where the airway becomes narrow or blocked during sleep.

However, not all breathing-related sleep problems are caused by airway obstruction.

In some cases, the problem lies deeper. It is not the airway that fails. It is the signal to breathe.

These conditions are less common but very important, especially in patients who do not improve with standard treatment for obstructive sleep apnea.

What Is Central Sleep Apnea?

Central sleep apnea is a condition in which the brain temporarily fails to send proper signals to the muscles that control breathing.

In simple terms, the body "forgets" to breathe for a few seconds.

Unlike obstructive sleep apnea, there is no blockage. The airway remains open, but there is no effort to breathe during that pause.

These episodes may occur multiple times during the night.

As a result, sleep becomes fragmented, and oxygen levels may fluctuate.

Patients often wake up feeling tired, even though they are not aware of these interruptions.

How It Differs From Obstructive Sleep Apnea

Understanding this difference is important.

In obstructive sleep apnea:

- The airway is blocked
- The body tries to breathe against the blockage

In central sleep apnea:

- The airway is open
- There is no breathing effort during the pause

The symptoms may look similar, such as fatigue or poor concentration, which is why proper testing is essential.

Doctor's Pearl

Not all sleep apnea is the same.
Correct diagnosis is the foundation of correct treatment.

Cheyne–Stokes Breathing – A Distinct Pattern

One specific pattern seen in central sleep apnea is called Cheyne–Stokes breathing.

In this pattern, breathing gradually becomes deeper and faster, then slows down, and then pauses. After the pause, the cycle repeats.

This pattern is often associated with heart failure or certain neurological conditions.

Recognizing this pattern is important because it may indicate an underlying medical problem that needs attention.

Sleep-Related Hypoventilation

Another important condition is sleep-related hypoventilation.

In this situation, breathing becomes too shallow during sleep.

The body does not get enough oxygen and does not remove enough carbon dioxide.

Patients may experience:

- Morning headaches
- Daytime fatigue
- Unrefreshing sleep

This condition is more common in:

- Obesity
- Chronic lung disease
- Neuromuscular disorders

Who Should Be Evaluated for These Conditions?

Not every patient with poor sleep needs evaluation for central sleep apnea or hypoventilation.

However, certain situations should raise concern.

You should consider evaluation if you have:

- Heart failure
- History of stroke
- Neurological conditions
- Persistent symptoms despite treatment for obstructive sleep apnea
- Use of opioid medications

In these cases, a detailed sleep study is often required.

Doctor's Pearl

If treatment for sleep apnea is not working, do not assume failure.
It may be the wrong diagnosis.

Why Accurate Diagnosis Is So Important

At first glance, all breathing-related sleep disorders may appear similar.

However, their treatment can be very different.

A treatment that works well for obstructive sleep apnea may not be effective for central sleep apnea.

Some patients may require different devices or treatment of the underlying medical condition.

This is why careful evaluation is essential.

Chapter Summary

Central sleep apnea occurs when the brain fails to send signals to breathe.

It differs from obstructive sleep apnea, where the airway is blocked.

Cheyne–Stokes breathing is a specific pattern linked to heart or neurological conditions.

Sleep-related hypoventilation involves shallow breathing and poor gas exchange.

These conditions are often associated with underlying medical problems.

Accurate diagnosis is essential for effective treatment.

Action Plan

- Do not ignore persistent fatigue despite treatment
- Inform your doctor about heart, lung, or neurological conditions
- Review medications that may affect breathing
- Follow through with recommended sleep studies
- Seek specialist evaluation when advised

Transition to Chapter 7

So far, we have focused on sleep disorders related to breathing.

However, not all sleep problems involve breathing.

In the next chapter, we will explore restless legs syndrome and periodic limb movements, conditions that disturb sleep through an uncomfortable urge to move.

CHAPTER 7: Restless Legs Syndrome – When the Body Refuses to Stay Still

A Different Kind of Sleep Problem

So far, we have discussed sleep problems related to breathing.

Restless Legs Syndrome, commonly called RLS, is very different.

Here, the difficulty is not in breathing and not always in falling asleep quickly. The problem comes from an uncomfortable sensation in the legs that creates a strong urge to move.

Patients often find it hard to describe.

They use words like:

- Crawling
- Tingling
- Pulling
- Inner restlessness

What they all share is a simple feeling.

"I cannot keep my legs still."

This sensation becomes worse when the body is at rest, especially in the evening or at bedtime.

Movement gives temporary relief, but the sensation soon returns.

As a result, falling asleep becomes difficult and sleep gets repeatedly disturbed.

Why Symptoms Are Worse at Night

One of the most characteristic features of RLS is its timing.

During the day, many patients feel normal or have only mild symptoms.

As evening approaches, the discomfort gradually increases.

At night, when the body becomes still, the sensation becomes more noticeable and more disturbing.

This is partly due to the body's internal rhythm. Certain brain chemicals that control movement fluctuate during the day.

Another reason is attention.

During the day, you are busy. At night, when everything is quiet, the sensation becomes more noticeable.

For many patients, bedtime becomes a struggle rather than a time of rest.

Doctor's Pearl

If your legs feel restless mainly at night and improve with movement, think of restless legs syndrome.

Common Causes and Contributing Factors

In some patients, no clear cause is found.

However, several important factors are well recognized.

Iron deficiency is one of the most common and treatable causes. Even when anemia is not present, low iron levels can trigger symptoms.

Chronic conditions may also play a role:

- Kidney disease
- Diabetes
- Peripheral nerve problems

Certain medications can worsen symptoms, including some antidepressants and antihistamines.

There is also a genetic component. RLS often runs in families.

With increasing age, symptoms may become more noticeable.

Periodic Limb Movement Disorder

Closely related to RLS is a condition called periodic limb movement disorder.

In this condition, the legs move involuntarily during sleep.

These movements are repetitive and may occur every few seconds to minutes.

Unlike RLS, the patient is usually not aware of these movements.

However, these repeated movements can disrupt sleep and reduce its quality.

Often, a bed partner notices these movements first.

In many cases, RLS and periodic limb movements occur together.

RESTLESS LEGS SYNDROME (RLS)

RLS is a condition that causes an uncomfortable urge to move your legs, usually when resting or trying to sleep.

WHAT HAPPENS

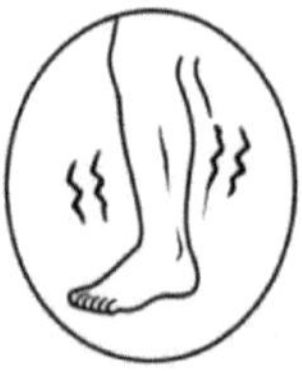

Unpleasant feelings in the legs – aching, tingling, crawling or throbbing.

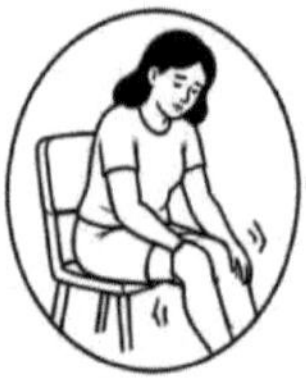

A strong urge to move the legs.

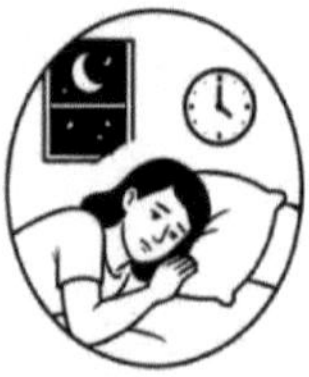

Symptoms start or get worse in the evening or at night.

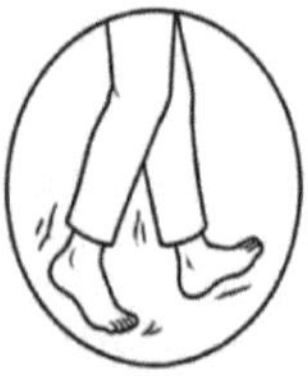

Relief with movement such as walking or stretching, but returns at rest.

WHY IT MATTERS

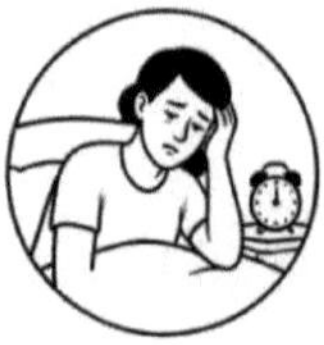

Makes it hard to fall asleep or stay asleep.

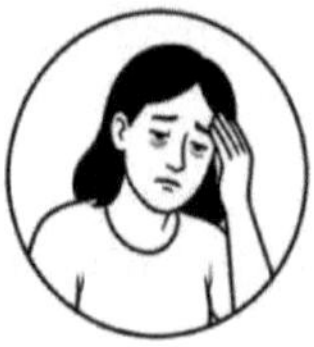

Causes daytime fatigue and poor concentration.

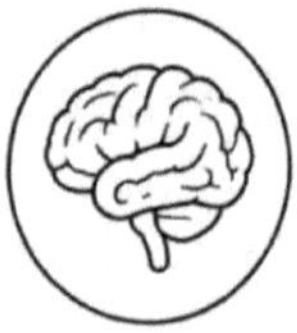

Affects mood and quality of life.

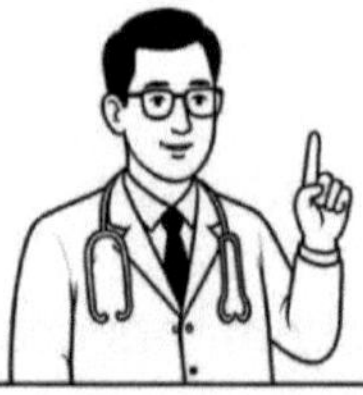

WHEN TO SEE A DOCTOR

See a doctor if:

- Symptoms are bothersome or affect your sleep
- Symptoms occur several times a week
- You feel tired during the day
- Home remedies do not help

RLS is treatable. Getting the right diagnosis and treatment can help you sleep better and feel better.

How RLS Affects Daily Life

Although the symptoms begin in the legs, their effects extend much further.

Difficulty falling asleep is common.

Even after falling asleep, repeated disturbances may interrupt normal sleep cycles.

Patients wake up feeling tired and unrefreshed.

During the day, they may experience:

- Fatigue
- Poor concentration
- Irritability

Over time, patients may begin to feel anxious about bedtime, expecting discomfort each night.

This creates an additional mental burden.

Doctor's Pearl

RLS is not just a leg problem.
It becomes a sleep problem, and then a daytime problem.

Managing Restless Legs Syndrome

The encouraging news is that RLS can often be managed effectively.

The first step is to identify and treat any underlying cause.

Checking iron levels is very important. Correcting deficiency can lead to significant improvement.

Lifestyle changes can help:

- Regular physical activity
- Consistent sleep schedule
- Reducing caffeine intake

Simple measures such as stretching, warm baths, or gentle massage before bedtime can provide relief.

In more severe cases, medications may be required.

These are selected carefully based on the patient's condition.

Chapter Summary

Restless Legs Syndrome causes an uncomfortable urge to move the legs, especially at rest and at night.

Symptoms are often described as crawling, tingling, or inner restlessness.

Iron deficiency and chronic conditions are common contributing factors.

Periodic limb movement disorder involves involuntary leg movements during sleep.

These conditions disrupt sleep and affect daytime functioning.

Effective treatment is available, especially when underlying causes are addressed.

Action Plan

- Pay attention to unusual sensations in your legs at night
- Ask your doctor to check iron levels
- Reduce caffeine intake
- Maintain a regular sleep schedule
- Try stretching or warm baths before bedtime
- Seek medical advice if symptoms persist

Transition to Chapter 8

Some sleep disorders make it difficult to fall asleep. Others disturb sleep after it begins.

There is another group where the main problem is excessive sleepiness during the day, even after a full night's sleep.

In the next chapter, we will explore narcolepsy and excessive daytime sleepiness.

CHAPTER 8: Narcolepsy and Excessive Daytime Sleepiness – When Staying Awake Becomes Difficult

Sleepiness That Goes Beyond Normal

Most of us feel sleepy at times.

After a poor night's sleep or a long day, it is natural to feel tired. A short rest or a good night's sleep usually corrects it.

Narcolepsy is very different.

Here, sleepiness is not occasional. It is persistent, overwhelming, and often unpredictable.

Patients often describe it in very simple and honest terms.

"Doctor, I cannot keep my eyes open."
"I sit for a few minutes, and I fall asleep."
"I feel sleepy even when I am talking to someone."

This is not laziness. It is not lack of discipline. It is a neurological condition that affects how the brain controls sleep and wakefulness.

What Exactly Is Narcolepsy?

Narcolepsy is a disorder in which the normal boundary between sleep and wakefulness becomes unstable.

Instead of having a clear separation between being awake and being asleep, elements of sleep can suddenly intrude into wakefulness.

This leads to episodes of excessive daytime sleepiness and, in some cases, sudden loss of muscle tone or dream-like experiences.

Even after what appears to be a full night's sleep, patients may still feel extremely sleepy during the day.

Key Symptoms You Should Recognize

The most important symptom is **excessive daytime sleepiness**.

Patients may fall asleep during routine activities such as reading, watching television, or sitting quietly. In some cases, sleep episodes may occur at inappropriate times, including while driving.

Some patients also experience **cataplexy**.

This is a sudden, brief loss of muscle strength triggered by strong emotions such as laughter, excitement, or anger. The person remains conscious but may feel weak or unable to move.

Another symptom is **sleep paralysis**.

This is a short period when a person cannot move or speak while falling asleep or waking up. It can be frightening but usually lasts only a few seconds to minutes.

Some patients also experience vivid dream-like sensations while falling asleep or waking up. These are known as hallucinations related to sleep transitions.

Not every patient has all of these symptoms, but recognizing them is important.

Doctor's Pearl

If sleepiness interferes with your daily activities despite adequate sleep, it is not normal fatigue.
It needs evaluation.

Why Narcolepsy Occurs

Narcolepsy is related to a problem in the brain's control of sleep and alertness.

In many patients, there is a deficiency of a chemical called hypocretin, which plays a key role in maintaining wakefulness.

When this system is affected, the brain cannot maintain stable wakefulness, and sleep intrudes unexpectedly.

The exact cause is not always clear. It may involve genetic factors and immune-related processes.

Impact on Daily Life and Safety

Narcolepsy can significantly affect daily life.

Patients often struggle to remain alert during important activities.

Work performance may decline. Learning and memory may be affected.

There is also a serious safety concern.

Sudden sleep episodes increase the risk of accidents, especially while driving or operating machinery.

Emotionally, patients may feel embarrassed or misunderstood. Because the condition is not widely recognized, they may be labeled as inattentive or unmotivated.

Understanding the condition helps remove this misunderstanding.

Doctor's Pearl

Narcolepsy is often misunderstood.
Recognizing it early can prevent unnecessary frustration and risk.

How Narcolepsy Is Diagnosed

Diagnosis requires careful evaluation.

A detailed history provides important clues, especially regarding daytime sleepiness and associated symptoms.

Sleep studies are usually required.

An overnight study may be followed by a daytime test that measures how quickly a person falls asleep and how often they enter dream sleep.

These tests help confirm the diagnosis and distinguish narcolepsy from other causes of sleepiness.

Management and Long-Term Care

Although narcolepsy cannot be completely cured, it can be effectively managed.

Treatment usually includes medications that improve alertness during the day.

Additional medications may be used if symptoms such as cataplexy are present.

Lifestyle adjustments are equally important.

Scheduled short naps during the day can help reduce sleepiness. Maintaining a regular sleep schedule is essential.

Patients should take precautions with activities that require full alertness until their condition is well controlled.

With proper management, many patients lead active and productive lives.

Chapter Summary

Narcolepsy is a neurological disorder characterized by excessive daytime sleepiness.

Patients may experience sudden sleep episodes despite adequate nighttime sleep.

Additional symptoms may include cataplexy, sleep paralysis, and vivid dream-like experiences.

The condition is related to abnormal regulation of sleep and wakefulness.

It can significantly affect daily life and safety.

With proper diagnosis and treatment, symptoms can be effectively managed.

NARCOLEPSY

Narcolepsy is a long-term brain disorder that affects the body's ability to control sleep and wakefulness.

KEY FEATURES

Excessive Daytime Sleepiness

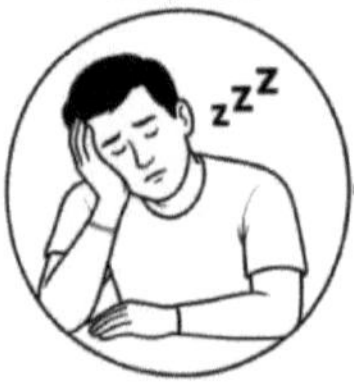

Overwhelming sleepiness during the day, even after a full night's sleep.

Sudden Sleep Attacks

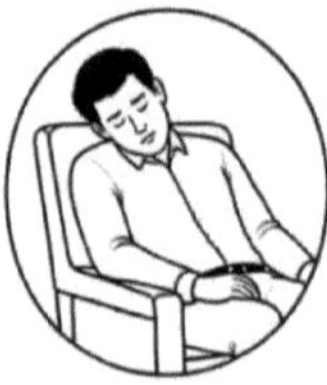

Falling asleep suddenly and without warning during activities.

Cataplexy

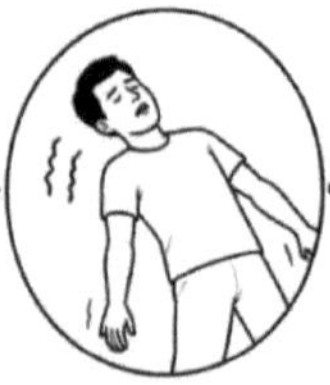

Sudden loss of muscle strength triggered by strong emotions such as laughter or surprise.

Disrupted Night Sleep

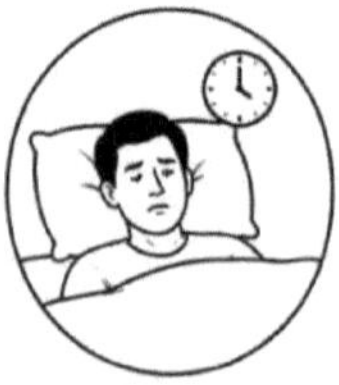

Frequent awakenings and non-restorative sleep at night.

OTHER POSSIBLE SYMPTOMS

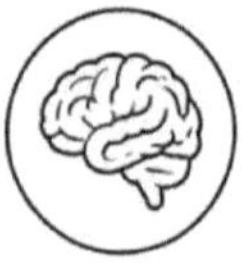

Sleep paralysis (temporary inability to move when falling asleep or waking up).

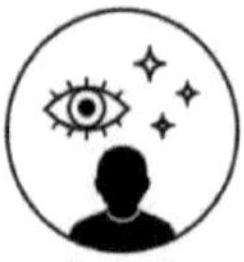

Hallucinations (seeing or sensing things that are not real while falling asleep or waking).

Symptoms can affect school, work, relationships and quality of life.

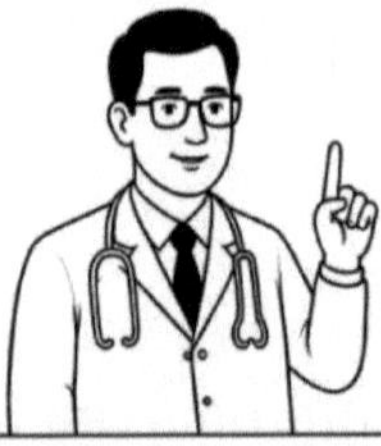

WHEN TO SEE A DOCTOR

See a doctor if you:

- Feel very sleepy during the day most days
- Fall asleep suddenly during activities
- Have episodes of muscle weakness with strong emotions
- Have trouble with nighttime sleep
- Snoring or other sleep problems may also be present

Narcolepsy is treatable. With the right diagnosis and treatment, you can live a better, more active life.

Action Plan

- Take persistent daytime sleepiness seriously
- Avoid high-risk activities if you feel excessively sleepy
- Maintain a regular sleep schedule
- Consider short, planned naps during the day
- Seek evaluation by a sleep specialist if symptoms are suggestive
- Follow treatment recommendations carefully

Transition to Chapter 9

So far, we have discussed sleep disorders related to breathing, movement, and daytime alertness.

There is another group of conditions where unusual behaviors occur during sleep.

In the next chapter, we will explore parasomnias, including sleepwalking, nightmares, and other sleep-related behaviors.

CHAPTER 9: Parasomnias – When Sleep Behaves in Unusual Ways

When Sleep Is Not Quiet and Still

Most people think of sleep as a calm and silent state.

You lie down, fall asleep, and remain still until morning.

But for some individuals, sleep can become surprisingly active.

Parasomnias are a group of conditions in which unusual behaviors, movements, or experiences occur during sleep.

These can range from simple talking to more complex actions such as walking, shouting, or acting out dreams.

Families are often the first to notice these changes.

A spouse may say, “You were talking loudly last night,” or “You suddenly sat up and looked frightened.”

These events can be confusing, and at times, frightening.

The important point is this. Not all parasomnias are dangerous, but some do require attention.

Common Types of Parasomnias

There are several types of parasomnias, and understanding them helps reduce unnecessary worry.

Sleep Talking
This is very common and usually harmless. It may occur occasionally or frequently, and in most cases, it does not need treatment.

Sleepwalking
In this condition, a person may sit up, walk around, or perform simple activities while still asleep. The person usually has no memory of the event the next morning.

Nightmares
These are vivid and disturbing dreams that wake the person. They are usually remembered clearly and often occur in the later part of the night.

Night Terrors
These are different from nightmares. The person may suddenly scream, sit up, or appear frightened but is not fully awake and usually does not remember the episode.

Each of these conditions has its own pattern and significance.

Doctor's Pearl

Not every unusual behavior during sleep is dangerous. But any behavior that causes fear, injury, or repeated disturbance needs attention.

REM Sleep Behavior Disorder – Acting Out Dreams

One important condition, especially in adults, is REM sleep behavior disorder.

Normally, during dream sleep, the body's muscles are relaxed. This prevents us from physically acting out dreams.

In this condition, that protective relaxation is lost.

As a result, the person may:

- Talk loudly
- Shout
- Move their arms or legs
- Act out dreams

In some cases, this can lead to injury to the patient or the bed partner.

This condition is important not only because of the risk of injury but also because it may be associated with certain neurological disorders.

Proper evaluation is essential.

Why Do Parasomnias Occur?

Parasomnias occur when the normal boundaries between sleep stages are disrupted.

In simple terms, the brain is partly asleep and partly awake at the same time.

This mixed state allows movements or behaviors to occur during sleep.

Several factors can increase the likelihood of parasomnias:

- Sleep deprivation
- Stress
- Irregular sleep schedules
- Alcohol use
- Certain medications

In children, parasomnias are relatively common and often improve with age.

In adults, especially when symptoms are new or worsening, they require more careful evaluation.

When Should You Be Concerned?

Many parasomnias are harmless.

However, certain situations require attention.

You should seek medical advice if:

- Episodes are frequent or increasing
- There is risk of injury
- Symptoms begin in adulthood
- Sleep quality is significantly affected
- Daytime functioning is impaired

Ignoring these signs may delay diagnosis and proper treatment.

Doctor's Pearl

New or worsening sleep behaviors in adults should never be ignored.
They may be the first sign of an underlying condition.

Managing Parasomnias Safely

Management depends on the type and severity of the condition.

In many cases, simple measures are effective.

Maintain a regular sleep schedule. Avoid sleep deprivation. Reduce stress.

Avoid alcohol, especially in the evening.

Safety is very important.

Make the sleeping environment safe:

- Remove sharp objects
- Ensure adequate space around the bed
- Consider precautions to prevent falls

In some cases, medications may be required. These are selected carefully based on the condition.

With proper care, most parasomnias can be managed effectively.

Chapter Summary

Parasomnias are unusual behaviors or experiences during sleep.

Common types include sleep talking, sleepwalking, nightmares, and night terrors.

REM sleep behavior disorder involves acting out dreams and may carry risk of injury.

Parasomnias occur due to disruption of normal sleep processes.

Many are harmless, but some require medical evaluation.

Safety and proper diagnosis are essential.

Action Plan

- Observe any unusual behaviors during sleep
- Ask family members for feedback
- Maintain a regular sleep schedule
- Reduce stress and avoid alcohol before bedtime
- Make your sleep environment safe
- Seek medical advice if symptoms are frequent or concerning

Transition to Chapter 10

So far, we have explored different types of sleep disorders.

Now, it is time to understand something even more important.

How do these sleep problems affect your overall health?

In the next chapter, we will explore how poor sleep impacts the heart, metabolism, and the entire body.

CHAPTER 10: How Poor Sleep Affects the Heart, Metabolism, and Overall Health

Sleep Is Deeply Connected to Your Health

Many people think of sleep as something that only affects how they feel the next day.

In reality, sleep has a much deeper impact.

It influences the heart, blood pressure, metabolism, weight, and even the risk of chronic diseases.

In my clinical practice, I have often seen patients struggle with conditions like high blood pressure or diabetes. They focus on medications, diet, and exercise, but sleep is often overlooked.

When sleep improves, many of these conditions become easier to manage.

That is why sleep should be seen as a central part of health, not a secondary one.

Sleep and Blood Pressure

During healthy sleep, the body enters a more relaxed state.

Blood pressure naturally falls. The heart rate slows down. This gives the cardiovascular system a chance to recover.

When sleep is disturbed, this natural drop in blood pressure does not occur properly.

In conditions like sleep apnea, repeated interruptions in breathing cause sudden increases in blood pressure and heart rate throughout the night.

Over time, this can lead to persistent high blood pressure.

Many patients with difficult-to-control hypertension show improvement once their sleep problem is treated.

Doctor's Pearl

If blood pressure is difficult to control, always think about sleep.
Sleep apnea is a common and often missed cause.

Sleep and Heart Disease

Poor sleep puts continuous stress on the heart.

Repeated awakenings, oxygen drops, and increased sympathetic activity place a burden on the cardiovascular system.

Over time, this increases the risk of:

- Coronary artery disease
- Heart attack
- Heart failure
- Irregular heart rhythms

Sleep apnea, in particular, has a strong association with these conditions.

Healthy sleep supports the heart. Poor sleep slowly damages it.

Sleep and Stroke Risk

The brain depends on stable blood flow and oxygen supply.

Repeated disturbances in sleep can affect blood vessels and increase the risk of stroke.

Fluctuations in blood pressure and oxygen levels, especially in sleep apnea, can damage the vascular system over time.

Sleep is now recognized as an important factor in stroke prevention.

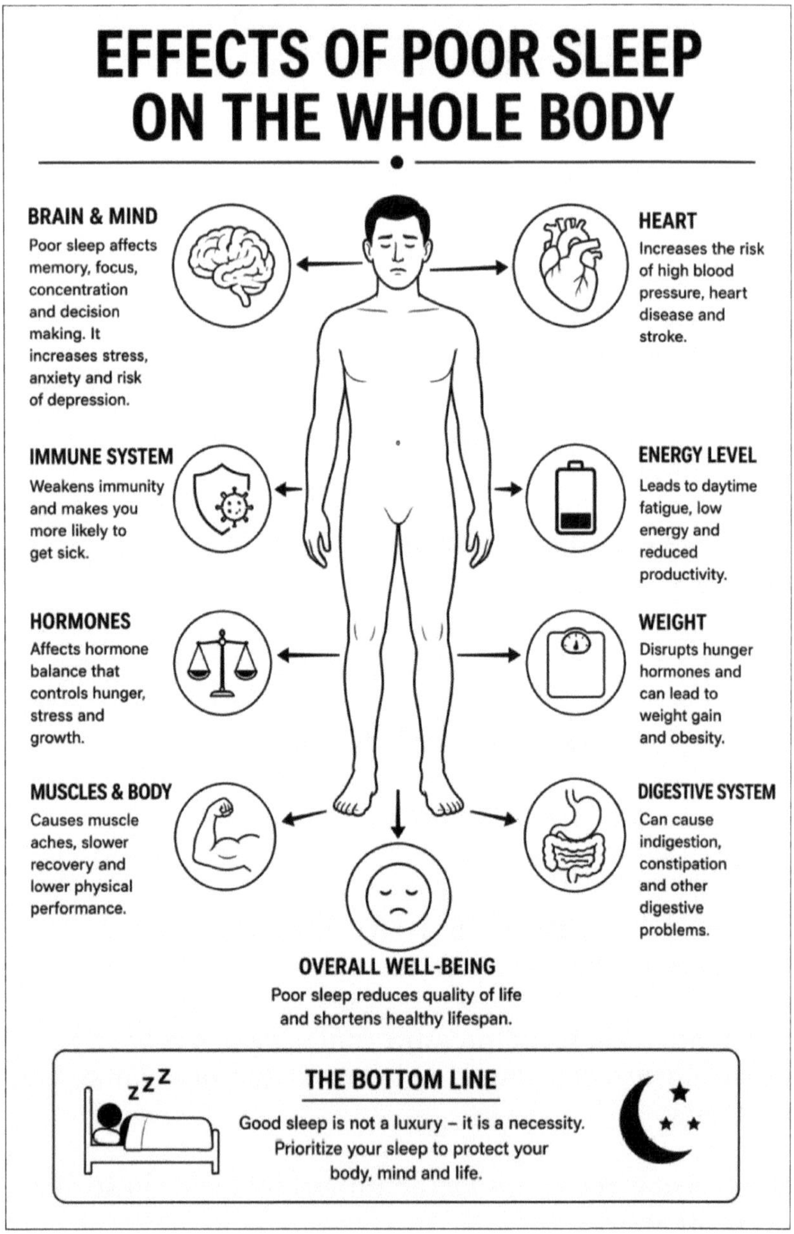
EFFECTS OF POOR SLEEP ON THE WHOLE BODY
BRAIN & MIND
Poor sleep affects memory, focus, concentration and decision making. It increases stress, anxiety and risk of depression.
HEART
Increases the risk of high blood pressure, heart disease and stroke.
IMMUNE SYSTEM
Weakens immunity and makes you more likely to get sick.
ENERGY LEVEL
Leads to daytime fatigue, low energy and reduced productivity.
HORMONES
Affects hormone balance that controls hunger, stress and growth.
WEIGHT
Disrupts hunger hormones and can lead to weight gain and obesity.
MUSCLES & BODY
Causes muscle aches, slower recovery and lower physical performance.
DIGESTIVE SYSTEM
Can cause indigestion, constipation and other digestive problems.
OVERALL WELL-BEING
Poor sleep reduces quality of life and shortens healthy lifespan.
zzz
THE BOTTOM LINE
Good sleep is not a luxury – it is a necessity. Prioritize your sleep to protect your body, mind and life.

Sleep and Weight Gain

There is a strong relationship between sleep and body weight.

When sleep is inadequate, hormones that control hunger and fullness become imbalanced.

Appetite increases, especially for high-calorie foods.

At the same time, low energy reduces motivation for physical activity.

This combination often leads to gradual weight gain.

Weight gain, in turn, can worsen sleep disorders such as sleep apnea, creating a cycle that becomes difficult to break.

Doctor's Pearl

Poor sleep increases appetite and reduces energy.
That combination almost always leads to weight gain.

Sleep and Diabetes

Sleep plays an important role in how the body regulates blood sugar.

Poor sleep reduces insulin sensitivity, meaning the body cannot use sugar effectively.

Over time, this increases the risk of developing type 2 diabetes.

In patients who already have diabetes, poor sleep makes blood sugar control more difficult.

Improving sleep often leads to better metabolic control.

Why Sleep Must Be a Priority

Traditionally, we focus on diet, exercise, and medications when managing health.

Sleep is often ignored.

But the reality is simple.

Without good sleep, the body cannot maintain balance.

Poor sleep increases the risk of multiple chronic conditions and makes existing conditions harder to manage.

The encouraging part is that sleep is something we can improve.

When sleep improves, it supports overall health in a powerful way.

Doctor's Pearl

You cannot achieve full health without good sleep. It is as important as diet and exercise.

Chapter Summary

Sleep has a major impact on the heart, blood pressure, and overall health.

Poor sleep is associated with hypertension, heart disease, and stroke.

Inadequate sleep contributes to weight gain and obesity.

Sleep plays a key role in blood sugar control and diabetes.

Sleep should be treated as a central pillar of long-term health.

Action Plan

- Take sleep seriously if you have high blood pressure or diabetes
- Pay attention to symptoms like snoring and fatigue
- Maintain a healthy weight
- Follow a regular sleep schedule
- Discuss sleep concerns during medical visits
- Seek evaluation if conditions are difficult to control

Transition to Chapter 11

We have seen how sleep affects the body.

Now it is time to understand how sleep affects the mind.

In the next chapter, we will explore how sleep influences memory, concentration, mood, and mental health.

CHAPTER 11: Sleep, the Brain, and Mental Well-Being

A Rested Mind Is a Clear Mind

In clinical practice, many patients come with concerns about memory, focus, or mood.

They often expect a discussion about medications, vitamins, or stress management.

But very often, when we explore their sleep, we find the real issue.

Sleep and brain function are closely connected.

When sleep is good, the mind feels clear, steady, and balanced. When sleep is poor, the mind feels slow, distracted, and easily overwhelmed.

This connection is powerful and often underestimated.

How Sleep Supports Memory and Learning

Every day, the brain is constantly absorbing information.

During sleep, especially deep sleep and dream sleep, the brain begins to organize and store this information.

Important details are strengthened. Less useful information is gradually filtered out.

Deep sleep helps consolidate factual memory. Dream sleep, also known as REM sleep, supports learning, creativity, and emotional processing.

When sleep is disturbed, this process becomes incomplete.

Patients often say:

- “I read something but cannot remember it”
- “My memory is not as sharp as before”

In many cases, the issue is not the brain itself. It is the quality of sleep.

Doctor’s Pearl

If your memory feels weak, do not immediately blame aging.
First, take a careful look at your sleep.

Sleep and Daily Concentration

A well-rested brain performs better.

After poor sleep, attention becomes unstable. It becomes harder to focus on tasks.

Small distractions become more noticeable. Reaction time slows. Decision-making becomes less reliable.

This has real-life consequences.

Work performance declines. Tasks take longer. Errors become more frequent.

In situations that require alertness, such as driving, poor sleep increases the risk of accidents.

A rested mind works efficiently. A tired mind struggles.

Sleep and Emotional Balance

Sleep plays a major role in emotional stability.

After good sleep, most people feel calmer and more balanced. They are better able to handle stress and respond thoughtfully.

After poor sleep, even small issues can feel overwhelming.

Patients often describe feeling:

- Irritable
- Anxious
- Easily upset

This is not surprising. Sleep helps regulate the emotional centers of the brain.

When sleep is disturbed, emotional control becomes weaker.

Doctor's Pearl

Poor sleep does not just affect your energy.
It changes how you react to life.

Sleep, Anxiety, and Depression

The relationship between sleep and mental health goes both ways.

Poor sleep can contribute to anxiety and depression.

At the same time, anxiety and depression can disturb sleep.

Patients with anxiety often report that their thoughts become more active at night.

Patients with depression may experience difficulty sleeping or may sleep longer but still feel tired.

Improving sleep is often a key part of managing these conditions.

Sleep and Long-Term Brain Health

As people grow older, concerns about memory and cognitive decline become more important.

Research suggests that poor sleep may contribute to long-term changes in brain health.

During sleep, the brain clears waste products that accumulate during the day.

When sleep is disturbed, this process may not work as efficiently.

Although sleep is only one factor, it is an important one.

Protecting sleep may help protect the brain.

Doctor's Pearl

Think of sleep as a nightly reset for your brain. Without it, the system slowly becomes overloaded.

Improving Mental Well-Being Through Better Sleep

One of the most encouraging things I see in practice is how quickly mental clarity improves when sleep improves.

Patients often report:

- Better focus
- Clearer thinking
- Improved mood
- Greater emotional stability

They feel more in control of their day and less overwhelmed.

Sleep is one of the simplest and most effective ways to support mental health.

Chapter Summary

Sleep is essential for memory, learning, and mental clarity.

Poor sleep reduces concentration and slows thinking.

Sleep plays a key role in emotional balance and mood regulation.

There is a strong connection between sleep and conditions like anxiety and depression.

Sleep may also influence long-term brain health.

Improving sleep can significantly enhance mental well-being.

Action Plan

- Pay attention to how sleep affects your focus and mood
- Maintain a regular sleep schedule
- Limit stimulating activities before bedtime
- Practice simple relaxation techniques
- Seek help if anxiety or depression affects your sleep
- Make sleep a priority for brain health

Transition to Chapter 12

You now understand how sleep affects both the body and the mind.

The next step is to understand how sleep problems are identified in medical practice.

In the next chapter, we will explore how doctors evaluate and diagnose sleep disorders.

CHAPTER 12: How Doctors Diagnose Sleep Disorders

Why Getting the Diagnosis Right Matters

In medicine, the success of treatment depends on one thing more than anything else.

That is the accuracy of the diagnosis.

Sleep problems are no different.

Many symptoms of poor sleep overlap with other conditions. Fatigue, low energy, poor concentration, and mood changes can come from many different causes.

If we do not look carefully, it is easy to treat the symptom and miss the real problem.

I have seen patients treated for stress or depression when the actual issue was sleep apnea. Others were taking medications for fatigue when the underlying problem was chronic insomnia.

Once the correct diagnosis is made, treatment becomes much more effective.

The Importance of a Detailed Sleep History

The most powerful diagnostic tool is not a machine. It is a careful conversation.

A detailed sleep history often provides the most important clues.

I usually begin with simple questions:

- How long does it take you to fall asleep?
- Do you wake up during the night?
- Do you feel refreshed in the morning?

Then we explore daytime symptoms:

- Do you feel sleepy during the day?
- Do you struggle to stay alert?
- Do you feel mentally clear?

Questions about snoring, choking, leg discomfort, or unusual behaviors during sleep help narrow down the possibilities.

A bed partner's observations are often very valuable. They may notice things the patient is not aware of.

A good history often points us in the right direction even before any tests are done.

Doctor's Pearl

In sleep medicine, listening carefully to the patient often provides more information than any machine.

HOW SLEEP DISORDERS ARE DIAGNOSED

Diagnosing a sleep disorder involves understanding your symptoms, sleep patterns and overall health.

1 MEDICAL HISTORY & DISCUSSION →

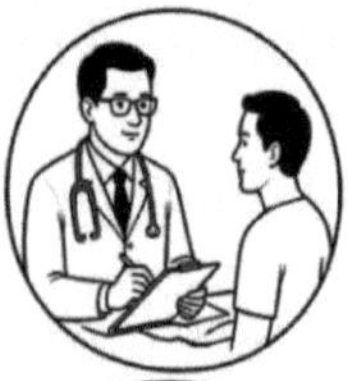

Your doctor will ask about your sleep problems, medical history, lifestyle, medications and family history.

2 SLEEP DIARY OR HISTORY →

You may be asked to keep a sleep diary to track your bed time, wake time, night awakenings and daytime sleepiness.

3 PHYSICAL EXAMINATION →

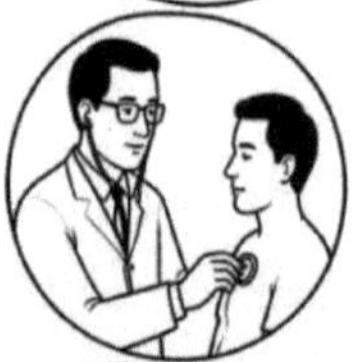

A physical exam helps identify any medical conditions that may be affecting your sleep.

4 SLEEP STUDY (POLYSOMNOGRAPHY) →

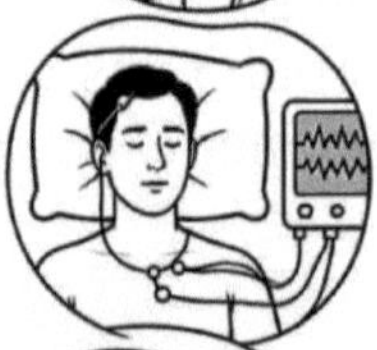

An overnight sleep study in a sleep lab records brain waves, breathing, oxygen levels, heart rate and body movements.

5 ADDITIONAL TESTS (IF NEEDED) →

Depending on your symptoms, tests like blood tests, actigraphy or multiple sleep latency test (MSLT) may be done.

Using Questionnaires to Guide Evaluation

To make the assessment more structured, doctors often use simple questionnaires.

These help measure symptoms such as daytime sleepiness or the likelihood of sleep apnea.

They do not provide a final diagnosis, but they help guide further evaluation.

They also help track progress over time.

The Role of a Sleep Diary

A sleep diary is a simple but very useful tool.

Patients record:

- Bedtime
- Time taken to fall asleep
- Night awakenings
- Wake-up time
- Daytime symptoms

Keeping a diary for one to two weeks often reveals patterns that are not obvious.

For example, irregular sleep timing or frequent awakenings may become clear only when recorded.

Some patients use wearable devices or apps. These can provide additional information, but they are not always fully accurate.

They should be used as a guide, not as a final answer.

Home Sleep Studies

For patients suspected of having sleep apnea, a home sleep study is often recommended.

This is done at home using a portable device.

It measures:

- Breathing patterns
- Oxygen levels
- Heart rate

Home studies are convenient and useful, especially for diagnosing moderate to severe obstructive sleep apnea.

However, they do not capture all aspects of sleep and may miss more complex conditions.

Polysomnography – A Detailed Sleep Study

When more detailed evaluation is needed, an in-lab sleep study is performed.

This is called polysomnography.

During this study, several body functions are monitored:

- Brain activity
- Breathing
- Oxygen levels
- Heart rate
- Body movements

This provides a comprehensive picture of sleep.

It is especially useful for diagnosing:

- Central sleep apnea
- Narcolepsy
- Parasomnias

Although spending a night in a sleep lab may feel unusual, the test is safe and very informative.

Doctor's Pearl

A sleep study does not disturb your sleep as much as you think.
The information it provides is often life-changing.

When to See a Sleep Specialist

Not every patient needs a specialist.

However, certain situations require expert evaluation.

You should consider seeing a specialist if:

- Symptoms are persistent or severe
- Diagnosis is unclear
- Initial treatment is not effective
- Complex conditions such as narcolepsy or unusual sleep behaviors are suspected

Early specialist evaluation can save time and prevent unnecessary treatments.

Chapter Summary

Accurate diagnosis is essential for effective treatment of sleep disorders.

A detailed sleep history is the most important first step.

Questionnaires and sleep diaries help identify patterns.

Home sleep studies are useful for diagnosing sleep apnea.

Polysomnography provides a comprehensive evaluation for complex cases.

Specialist consultation is important when needed.

Action Plan

- Keep a sleep diary for one to two weeks
- Note symptoms such as snoring and daytime sleepiness
- Discuss sleep concerns openly with your doctor
- Follow recommended tests
- Do not rely only on apps or devices
- Seek specialist care when needed

Transition to Chapter 13

Once a sleep problem is clearly identified, the next step is treatment.

In many cases, the most effective treatment does not begin with medicines or devices.

It begins with simple, natural changes in daily habits.

In the next chapter, we will explore natural ways to improve sleep.

CHAPTER 13: Natural Ways to Improve Sleep

Start With What Works Naturally

When patients struggle with sleep, many expect a prescription.

But in my experience, the most powerful improvements often begin without medication.

They begin with daily habits.

Sleep is not something we can force. It is something we can support.

When we align our routine with how the body naturally works, sleep begins to improve on its own.

This chapter focuses on simple, practical steps that can make a meaningful difference.

Sleep Hygiene – The Foundation of Good Sleep

The term “sleep hygiene” simply means habits that support healthy sleep.

The most important habit is a **consistent sleep schedule**.

Going to bed and waking up at the same time every day helps train your internal clock. Even small variations can disturb this rhythm.

Your sleeping environment also matters.

A good bedroom should be:

- Quiet
- Dark
- Comfortably cool

Use the bed only for sleep.

Avoid watching television, using your phone, or working in bed. This helps the brain associate the bed with sleep rather than activity.

Doctor’s Pearl

Your body loves routine.
The more regular your schedule, the easier sleep becomes.

Food, Caffeine, and Alcohol

What you consume, especially in the evening, has a strong effect on sleep.

Caffeine is one of the most common disruptors. It can remain in the body for several hours. Even afternoon intake can affect nighttime sleep.

Heavy meals late in the evening can cause discomfort and interfere with sleep.

Alcohol is often misunderstood.

It may help you fall asleep faster, but it disrupts deeper sleep and causes frequent awakenings later in the night.

Making small changes in these habits can lead to noticeable improvement.

Exercise and Daily Activity

Regular physical activity is one of the most effective ways to improve sleep.

It helps the body feel naturally tired at night and reduces stress.

However, timing matters.

Moderate exercise during the day improves sleep. Very intense exercise close to bedtime may delay sleep in some individuals.

Even simple activities like walking can be helpful.

NATURAL WAYS TO IMPROVE SLEEP

Simple daily habits for better, deeper sleep.

1. KEEP A SLEEP SCHEDULE

Go to bed and wake up at the same time every day, even on weekends.

2. GET NATURAL DAYLIGHT

Spend time outside in the morning. It helps regulate your body clock.

3. EXERCISE REGULARLY

Aim for at least 30 minutes of activity most days. Avoid intense exercise close to bedtime.

4. LIMIT CAFFEINE & ALCOHOL

Avoid caffeine in the afternoon and evening. Limit alcohol, especially before bed.

5. EAT LIGHT AT NIGHT

Avoid heavy, spicy or sugary foods close to bedtime. A light snack is okay if you're hungry.

6. REDUCE SCREEN TIME

Limit screens at least 1 hour before bed. The blue light can make it harder to fall asleep.

7. CREATE A SLEEP FRIENDLY ENVIRONMENT

Keep your room cool, dark and quiet. Make your bed comfortable and clutter-free.

8. MANAGE STRESS & RELAX

Try deep breathing, meditation, journaling or gentle stretching before bed.

9. TRY SOOTHING NATURAL REMEDIES

Herbal teas (chamomile, lemon balm), warm milk, magnesium or lavender aromatherapy may promote relaxation.

10. ESTABLISH A BEDTIME ROUTINE

Do the same relaxing activities each night to signal your body it's time to wind down.

11. STAY HYDRATED (EARLIER IN THE DAY)

Drink enough water during the day, but limit fluids 1–2 hours before bed to avoid nighttime awakenings.

12. KEEP IT CONSISTENT

Consistency is key. Small daily habits lead to better sleep and better health.

**Better sleep starts with small, natural choices every day.
Your body and mind will thank you.**

Light Exposure and the Body Clock

Light plays a powerful role in regulating sleep.

Morning sunlight signals the body to stay alert and active.

As evening approaches and light decreases, the body begins to prepare for sleep.

Late exposure to artificial light, especially from screens, interferes with this process.

Reducing screen use before bedtime helps the body produce melatonin, the hormone that supports sleep.

Doctor's Pearl

Morning light wakes up your body clock.
Evening darkness prepares it for sleep.

Calming the Mind Before Bedtime

For many patients, the biggest barrier to sleep is not the body, but the mind.

At night, when everything becomes quiet, thoughts become louder.

Worries, plans, and unfinished tasks begin to surface.

A calming routine before bedtime can help.

This may include:

- Reading something light
- Listening to soft music
- Practicing slow breathing

Writing down your thoughts earlier in the evening can also help reduce mental activity at bedtime.

A Simple Evening Routine

A predictable routine helps signal the body that it is time to sleep.

About an hour before bedtime:

- Reduce stimulation
- Dim the lights
- Avoid stressful or emotional activities

If you cannot fall asleep, do not remain in bed feeling frustrated.

Get up, go to another room, and do a quiet activity until you feel sleepy.

This helps prevent the bed from becoming associated with wakefulness.

Doctor's Pearl

Do not fight sleep.
Create the right conditions, and sleep will come.

Chapter Summary

Healthy sleep begins with consistent daily habits.

A regular sleep schedule is one of the most important factors.

The sleep environment should be quiet, dark, and comfortable.

Caffeine, heavy meals, and alcohol can disrupt sleep.

Exercise and light exposure support the body's natural rhythm.

A calm bedtime routine helps prepare the mind for sleep.

Action Plan

- Fix a consistent sleep and wake time
- Reduce caffeine in the afternoon and evening

- Limit screen use before bedtime
- Keep your bedroom quiet, dark, and comfortable
- Develop a simple bedtime routine
- Stay consistent with these habits

Transition to Chapter 14

For many people, these natural steps bring significant improvement.

However, in chronic insomnia, deeper patterns of thought and behavior often keep the problem going.

In the next chapter, we will explore Cognitive Behavioral Therapy for Insomnia, one of the most effective long-term treatments.

CHAPTER 14: Cognitive Behavioral Therapy for Insomnia – Retraining the Mind for Better Sleep

Looking Beyond Quick Fixes

When sleep becomes a long-standing problem, many patients naturally look for a quick solution.

A pill feels simple. It promises immediate relief.

And in some situations, it does help for a short time.

But chronic insomnia is rarely solved by a quick fix.

In my experience, lasting improvement comes from understanding and correcting the patterns that keep insomnia going.

This is where Cognitive Behavioral Therapy for Insomnia, often called CBT-I, becomes very important.

What Is CBT-I and Why It Works

CBT-I is a structured, practical approach that helps restore natural sleep.

It does not rely on medication.

Instead, it works by changing:

- Sleep habits
- Thought patterns
- Behaviors around bedtime

Insomnia is not just a nighttime problem. It becomes a learned pattern.

A few bad nights create worry. Worry creates tension. The bed becomes associated with frustration.

CBT-I breaks this cycle.

It helps the mind and body return to a healthier pattern.

Doctor's Pearl

Insomnia is often learned over time.
The good news is that it can also be unlearned.

Rebuilding the Link Between Bed and Sleep

One of the most important steps in CBT-I is called **stimulus control**.

The idea is simple.

The bed should mean sleep, not wakefulness.

If you spend long periods awake in bed, your brain begins to associate the bed with thinking, worrying, and frustration.

Stimulus control corrects this.

You go to bed only when you feel sleepy.

If you cannot sleep within a reasonable time, you get out of bed and do something quiet until you feel sleepy again.

Over time, the brain relearns that the bed is a place for sleep.

Using Time in Bed More Effectively

Many patients try to compensate for poor sleep by spending more time in bed.

This often makes sleep lighter and more fragmented.

CBT-I uses a different approach.

Time in bed is adjusted to match actual sleep time more closely.

This helps build a stronger natural drive for sleep.

As sleep improves, time in bed is gradually increased.

This step is done carefully and gradually.

Working With Thoughts, Not Against Them

Thoughts play a major role in insomnia.

Common thoughts include:

- "I will not be able to function tomorrow"
- "Something is wrong with my sleep"

These thoughts increase anxiety, which makes sleep more difficult.

CBT-I helps patients recognize these patterns and respond to them in a more balanced way.

The goal is not to force positive thinking.

It is to reduce unnecessary worry and create a calmer mental state.

Doctor's Pearl

Sleep improves when the mind becomes less anxious about sleep itself.

COGNITIVE BEHAVIORAL THERAPY FOR INSOMNIA (CBT-I)

A proven, non-medication approach that helps you identify and change thoughts and behaviors that cause sleep problems.

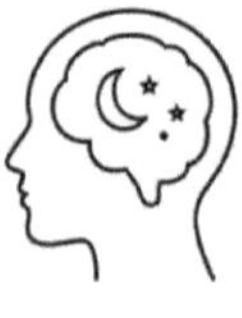

WHAT IS CBT-I?

CBT-I (Cognitive Behavioral Therapy for Insomnia) helps you develop healthier sleep habits and change unhelpful thoughts and behaviors that keep you from sleeping well.

THE CORE COMPONENTS OF CBT-I

1 SLEEP EDUCATION

Learn about sleep, how it works and what affects it.

2 SLEEP RESTRICTION

Limit time in bed to match your actual sleep time, then gradually increase it.

3 STIMULUS CONTROL

Strengthen the link between bed and sleep. Use bed only for sleep and intimacy.

4 COGNITIVE RESTRUCTURING

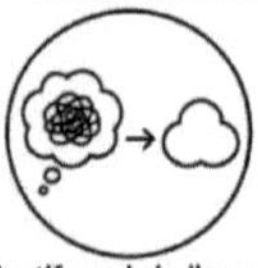

Identify and challenge unhelpful thoughts and worries about sleep.

5 RELAXATION TECHNIQUES

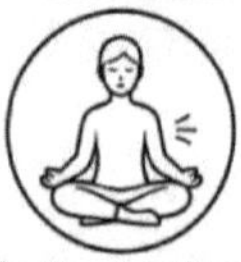

Use deep breathing, progressive muscle relaxation or mindfulness to reduce tension and stress.

6 SLEEP HYGIENE IMPROVEMENT

Build healthy daily habits that support better sleep (routine, light, exercise, caffeine, screens, etc.).

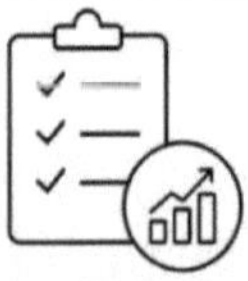

BENEFITS OF CBT-I

- ✓ Improves sleep quality and duration
- ✓ Reduces time to fall asleep and nighttime awakenings
- ✓ Improves daytime alertness, mood and functioning
- ✓ Long-lasting results without medication

Practical Tools That Make a Difference

CBT-I is not just theory. It includes simple, practical tools.

A fixed wake-up time is one of the most important anchors for the body clock.

Avoiding long periods of wakefulness in bed helps break the insomnia cycle.

A short sleep diary helps track patterns without creating stress.

Relaxation techniques such as slow breathing or quiet reading can help calm the mind.

These steps may appear simple, but they are very effective when practiced consistently.

Accessing CBT-I in Real Life

CBT-I can be delivered in different ways.

Some patients work with trained therapists over several sessions.

There are also structured online programs that guide patients step by step.

What matters most is consistency.

Patients who follow the program regularly tend to see the best results.

Doctor's Pearl

CBT-I requires patience, but it offers long-term results without dependence on medication.

Chapter Summary

CBT-I is a structured, non-drug approach to treating insomnia.

It works by changing behaviors and thought patterns related to sleep.

Key steps include rebuilding the association between bed and sleep and adjusting time in bed.

Managing anxious thoughts is an important part of treatment.

With consistent practice, CBT-I can provide long-term improvement.

Action Plan

- Fix a consistent wake-up time
- Go to bed only when you feel sleepy

- Avoid staying awake in bed for long periods
- Practice a calming bedtime routine
- Keep a simple sleep diary
- Stay patient and consistent

Transition to Chapter 15

CBT-I provides a strong, long-term solution for insomnia.

However, there are situations where medications may be helpful, especially for short-term support.

In the next chapter, we will discuss sleep medications, how they work, and how to use them safely.

CHAPTER 15: Medicines for Sleep – When to Use Them and How to Use Them Safely

A Practical and Balanced Approach

When patients struggle with sleep, one of the first questions they ask is very simple.

"Doctor, can you give me something to help me sleep?"

It is a reasonable question.

Medicines can help. But they must be used carefully, thoughtfully, and for the right reasons.

In earlier chapters, we discussed lifestyle changes and behavioral therapies. These form the foundation of good sleep.

Medications are usually considered when:

- Sleep problems are severe
- Symptoms are persistent
- Daily functioning is significantly affected

The goal is not just to produce sleep for a few nights. The goal is to restore healthy, natural sleep.

Types of Sleep Medications

There is no single medication that works for everyone.

Different medicines are used depending on the type of sleep problem.

Some help you fall asleep faster.
Some help you stay asleep longer.
Some help regulate the sleep–wake cycle.

In certain situations, medications used for anxiety or depression may also improve sleep.

For conditions like restless legs syndrome or narcolepsy, specific medications are used to treat the underlying problem.

The choice always depends on the individual patient.

Doctor's Pearl

There is no "one best sleeping pill."
The right medicine depends on the patient, not the label.

When Medications Can Be Helpful

Used appropriately, medications can provide meaningful relief.

Short-term insomnia, such as during stress or illness, may respond well to a brief course of medication.

Sometimes, improving sleep for a few nights helps break the cycle of anxiety around sleep.

Medications may also be used while starting behavioral therapy, providing temporary support until long-term strategies begin to work.

The key is careful and time-limited use.

Understanding the Limitations

It is important to understand what sleep medications can and cannot do.

Most medications do not correct the underlying cause of insomnia. They mainly help control symptoms.

Over time, their effectiveness may decrease. This is known as tolerance.

Some patients begin to feel that they cannot sleep without medication. This is known as dependence.

These risks do not mean that medications should be avoided completely.

They mean that medications should be used wisely.

SLEEP MEDICINES:
TYPES, USES & CONSIDERATIONS

Sleep medicines can help in the short term or for specific sleep disorders. They should be used under a doctor's guidance.

TYPES OF SLEEP MEDICINES

TYPE	EXAMPLES	USES
1. SEDATIVE–HYPNOTICS (Non-benzodiazepine) Help you fall asleep faster and stay asleep.	• Zolpidem • Eszopiclone • Zaleplon	Short-term treatment of insomnia.
2. BENZODIAZEPINES Slow brain activity and promote relaxation.	• Temazepam • Lorazepam • Triazolam	Short-term insomnia or severe anxiety related to sleep.
3. MELATONIN RECEPTOR AGONISTS Mimic melatonin, the hormone that regulates sleep–wake cycle.	• Ramelteon	Help with sleep onset insomnia.
4. ANTIDEPRESSANTS Affect brain chemicals to improve sleep.	• Trazodone • Amitriptyline • Doxepin (low dose)	Insomnia with depression, chronic pain or anxiety.
5. ANTIHISTAMINES Cause drowsiness by blocking histamine.	• Diphenhydramine • Doxylamine	Occasional short-term use for mild insomnia or allergies.
6. WAKE-PROMOTING AGENTS Help you stay awake during the day.	• Modafinil • Armodafinil • Solriamfetol	Daytime sleepiness caused by conditions like narcolepsy or sleep apnea.

IMPORTANT THINGS TO KNOW

- Use the lowest effective dose for the shortest time.
- May cause drowsiness, dizziness or dependence.
- Avoid alcohol and driving after taking these medicines.
- Not a substitute for good sleep habits and routine.
- Always follow your doctor's advice.

TIPS FOR SAFE USE

- Take only when you can sleep for 7–8 hours.
- Take 30–60 minutes before bedtime (as directed).
- Do not stop suddenly if used for a long time.
- Regularly review the need for continuing the medicine with your doctor.
- Report any side effects to your doctor.

MEDICINES CAN HELP, BUT BETTER SLEEP STARTS WITH HEALTHY HABITS AND ROUTINES.

Doctor's Pearl

Sleep medicines can support sleep, but they cannot replace healthy sleep habits.

Possible Side Effects and Risks

Like all medications, sleep medicines can have side effects.

Common ones include:

- Daytime drowsiness
- Dizziness
- Reduced alertness

In older adults, these effects can increase the risk of falls.

Some patients may experience memory issues or unusual behaviors during sleep.

The exact risks vary depending on the medication and the individual.

This is why proper medical guidance is essential.

Special Considerations in Older Adults

Older adults need extra caution when using sleep medications.

The body processes drugs more slowly with age.

This increases the risk of:

- Confusion
- Imbalance
- Falls

For this reason, lower doses are used, and some medications are avoided altogether.

Non-drug approaches become even more important in this group.

Common Mistakes to Avoid

Over the years, I have seen certain patterns that can create problems.

Some patients increase the dose on their own when the effect seems less.

Others continue medications for long periods without review.

Some rely entirely on medication and ignore sleep habits.

These approaches often lead to more difficulty over time.

Doctor's Pearl

If you need more medicine over time, the problem is not improving.
It needs a different approach.

A Balanced, Long-Term Strategy

The most effective approach combines different methods.

Lifestyle changes, behavioral therapy, and medications when needed can work together.

The goal is to:

- Use medication when necessary
- Use the lowest effective dose
- Limit duration when possible
- Gradually reduce dependence

With this balanced approach, patients can benefit from medications without becoming dependent on them.

Chapter Summary

Sleep medications can be helpful but are not the first-line treatment for most sleep problems.

Different types of medications are used depending on the condition.

They are most useful for short-term relief or specific situations.

Limitations include tolerance and dependence.

Side effects must be considered, especially in older adults.

Medications should be part of a broader treatment plan.

Action Plan

- Use sleep medications only when clearly needed
- Follow your doctor's instructions carefully
- Do not increase the dose on your own
- Watch for side effects
- Combine medication use with lifestyle changes
- Plan for gradual reduction when appropriate

Transition to Chapter 16

While medications have a role, they are not the primary treatment for all sleep disorders.

In conditions like sleep apnea, the most effective treatment often involves devices that support breathing during sleep.

In the next chapter, we will explore CPAP, BiPAP, and other devices that can significantly improve sleep and health.

CHAPTER 16: CPAP, BiPAP, and Other Devices – Treatments That Can Transform Sleep

When Treatment Is Not a Pill

When patients hear that they may need a machine to sleep, the first reaction is often hesitation.

It feels unfamiliar. Sometimes even intimidating.

Many ask, "Doctor, do I really need this?"

In my experience, once patients understand how these devices work, and more importantly, once they begin to feel the benefits, their hesitation slowly disappears.

For conditions like sleep apnea, these devices are often the most effective treatment.

What CPAP Really Does

The most commonly used device is called CPAP, which stands for Continuous Positive Airway Pressure.

I usually explain it in a simple way.

CPAP delivers a gentle stream of air through a mask worn over the nose or mouth. This air does not breathe for you.

Instead, it keeps your airway open.

During sleep, the throat muscles relax. In some people, this causes the airway to narrow or collapse.

CPAP acts like a soft support that prevents this collapse.

As a result:

- Breathing remains steady
- Oxygen levels stay normal
- Sleep becomes deeper and less interrupted

Doctor's Pearl

CPAP does not force you to breathe.
It simply keeps the airway open so your body can breathe naturally.

The First Few Nights – What Patients Experience

Starting CPAP is often the most challenging part.

Wearing a mask feels unusual at first. Some patients feel uncomfortable or slightly anxious.

Others notice dryness in the nose or mouth.

It is important to understand that this phase is temporary.

The body and mind need time to adjust.

Patients who continue usually begin to notice improvement:

- Better sleep quality
- Reduced daytime fatigue
- Improved energy

This adjustment period is a normal part of the process.

Common Problems and Simple Solutions

Most CPAP-related issues can be managed with simple adjustments.

If the mask feels uncomfortable, changing the size or type often helps. There are several designs available.

If dryness occurs, a humidifier can improve comfort.

If the pressure feels too strong, many devices allow gradual pressure increase.

If anxiety is present, practicing with the mask during the day can help.

The key is to address problems early rather than stopping treatment.

Doctor's Pearl

Do not give up on CPAP too early.
Most problems have simple solutions.

Other Device Options

CPAP is the most common treatment, but it is not the only option.

BiPAP (Bilevel Positive Airway Pressure)
This provides different pressures for inhalation and exhalation. It may be more comfortable for some patients.

Oral Appliances
These are worn like a mouthguard. They help keep the airway open by adjusting the position of the jaw.

Positional Therapy
Some patients have worse apnea when sleeping on their back. Changing sleep position may help.

The best option depends on the individual patient.

SLEEP DEVICES:
CPAP, BIPAP & OTHER DEVICES

Sleep devices help treat sleep disorders by keeping your airways open, improving breathing and supporting better sleep.

POSITIVE AIRWAY PRESSURE (PAP) DEVICES

1. CPAP (CONTINUOUS POSITIVE AIRWAY PRESSURE)

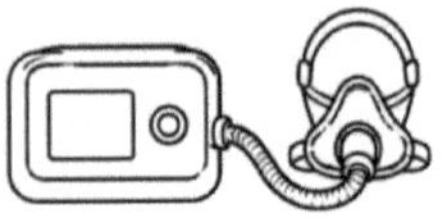

Delivers a constant, steady air pressure through a mask to keep airways open during sleep.

USES:
- Obstructive Sleep Apnea (OSA)

2. BIPAP (BILEVEL POSITIVE AIRWAY PRESSURE)

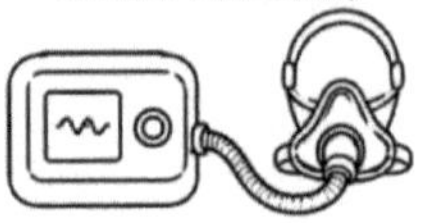

Delivers two levels of pressure—higher when you inhale and lower when you exhale—for easier breathing.

USES:
- Sleep apnea
- COPD
- Hypoventilation syndromes

3. APAP (AUTOMATIC POSITIVE AIRWAY PRESSURE)

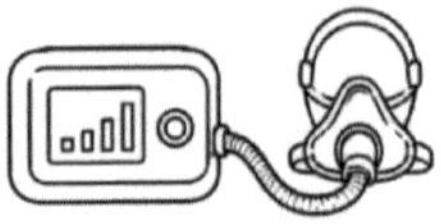

Automatically adjusts pressure throughout the night based on your breathing needs.

USES:
- Obstructive Sleep Apnea (OSA)

OTHER SLEEP DEVICES

4. ORAL APPLIANCE (MANDIBULAR ADVANCEMENT DEVICE)

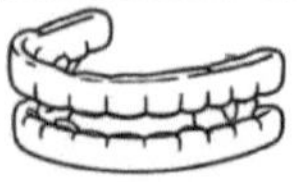

A custom-fit device worn in the mouth that repositions the jaw and tongue to keep the airway open.

USES:
- Mild to moderate OSA
- Snoring

5. POSITIONAL THERAPY DEVICES

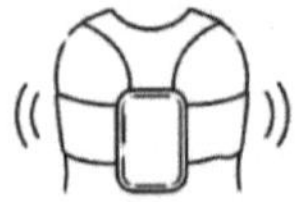

Helps prevent sleeping on the back, which can worsen sleep apnea in some people.

USES:
- Positional Obstructive Sleep Apnea

6. NASAL EXPIRATORY POSITIVE AIRWAY PRESSURE (EPAP) DEVICES

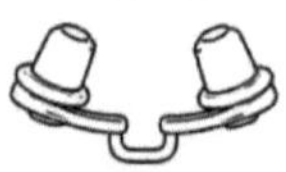

Small valves placed over the nostrils create back pressure when exhaling to keep airways open.

USES:
- Mild OSA
- Snoring

7. HYPOGLOSSAL NERVE STIMULATOR (INSPIRE® THERAPY)

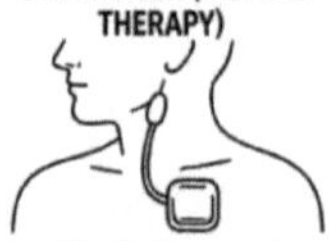

A small implant that stimulates the nerve controlling tongue movement to keep the airway open during sleep.

USES:
- Moderate to severe OSA in adults who cannot use CPAP

GENERAL BENEFITS

- Improve breathing and oxygen levels during sleep
- Reduce snoring and nighttime awakenings
- Improve daytime alertness, mood and quality of life
- Lower risk of heart and other health problems

TIPS FOR USING SLEEP DEVICES

- Use your device every night for the entire sleep time.
- Follow your doctor's instructions and device settings.
- Keep your device and accessories clean.
- Replace masks, filters and parts as recommended.
- Regular follow-up ensures the best results.

The right device, used consistently, can make a big difference in your sleep, health and overall well-being.

Always consult your sleep specialist to find the best option for you.

Why Consistency Is So Important

The effectiveness of these devices depends on regular use.

Using CPAP occasionally does not provide full benefit.

Patients who use the device every night often experience significant improvement.

Over time, this may also help improve blood pressure and overall health.

Consistency turns treatment into results.

What Patients Often Notice

One of the most rewarding parts of treating sleep apnea is seeing the change in patients.

Many say they feel like a different person.

They wake up refreshed. They have more energy. Their thinking becomes clearer.

Family members also notice improvement. Snoring decreases or disappears. Sleep becomes more peaceful for everyone.

These changes motivate patients to continue treatment.

Doctor's Pearl

When CPAP works, patients often say, "I did not realize how tired I was before."

Chapter Summary

CPAP is a device that keeps the airway open during sleep using gentle air pressure.

It is one of the most effective treatments for obstructive sleep apnea.

Initial discomfort is common but usually improves with time.

Most problems can be managed with simple adjustments.

Other options include BiPAP, oral appliances, and positional therapy.

Regular use is essential for full benefit.

Action Plan

- Give yourself time to adjust to CPAP
- Work with your provider to find a comfortable mask
- Use the device every night
- Address problems early
- Stay consistent with treatment

- Keep follow-up appointments

Transition to Chapter 17

For many patients, these devices provide excellent results.

However, some situations require additional or specialized approaches.

In the next chapter, we will explore advanced treatments and special situations in sleep disorders.

CHAPTER 17: Advanced Treatments and Special Situations

When Standard Treatment Is Not Enough

For many patients, sleep improves with lifestyle changes, behavioral therapy, medications when needed, or devices like CPAP.

However, there is a smaller group of patients in whom these standard approaches do not provide complete relief.

This can be frustrating.

But it is important to understand that this does not mean the problem cannot be treated. It simply means we need a more individualized approach.

In such situations, careful evaluation, patience, and a combination of strategies often lead to better outcomes.

Surgical Options in Sleep Apnea

Surgery is not the first step in treating sleep apnea.

However, in selected patients, it can be helpful.

Some procedures aim to remove or reduce excess tissue in the throat to widen the airway.

Others correct structural problems such as:

- A deviated nasal septum
- Enlarged tonsils
- Narrow jaw structure

In more complex cases, surgery may involve repositioning parts of the jaw to increase airway space.

The decision to proceed with surgery depends on:

- Severity of sleep apnea
- Patient's anatomy
- Response to other treatments

A detailed discussion with a specialist is essential.

Doctor's Pearl

Surgery is not for everyone.
The right patient selection makes all the difference.

Newer and Emerging Therapies

Advances in sleep medicine have introduced new treatment options.

One such option is **nerve stimulation therapy**.

In this approach, a small device is implanted to stimulate the muscles that help keep the airway open during sleep.

This may be considered in patients who cannot tolerate CPAP.

Technology is also improving existing devices, making them more comfortable and easier to use.

These developments are expanding the range of effective treatments.

Sleep in Older Adults

Sleep patterns naturally change with age.

Sleep may become lighter. Night awakenings may increase.

However, poor sleep should not be accepted as a normal part of aging.

Older adults often have multiple factors affecting sleep:

- Medical conditions
- Medications
- Reduced physical activity
- Irregular routines

They are also more sensitive to the side effects of sleep medications.

Careful evaluation and individualized treatment are especially important in this group.

Doctor's Pearl

Aging changes sleep patterns, but it should not reduce sleep quality.

Sleep and Chronic Medical Conditions

Sleep and chronic illness often influence each other.

Conditions such as:

- Heart disease
- Lung disease
- Diabetes
- Neurological disorders

can disturb sleep.

At the same time, poor sleep can worsen these conditions.

For example:

- Untreated sleep apnea can worsen blood pressure
- Poor sleep can affect blood sugar control

Managing sleep as part of overall health care often leads to better results.

Shift Work and Irregular Schedules

Modern life does not always follow a natural sleep pattern.

People who work night shifts or rotating schedules may develop **shift work sleep disorder**.

In this condition, the body's internal clock is out of sync with work and sleep timing.

This leads to:

- Poor sleep quality
- Daytime fatigue
- Reduced alertness

Frequent travel across time zones can cause **jet lag**, which temporarily disrupts sleep.

Planning becomes very important in these situations.

Doctor's Pearl

When your schedule conflicts with your body clock, sleep will suffer.
Planning helps reduce the damage.

Managing Special Situations

In these more complex situations, management requires flexibility.

Some helpful strategies include:

- Gradually adjusting sleep schedules
- Using light exposure strategically
- Maintaining consistent routines when possible
- Prioritizing sleep even with a busy schedule

In some cases, medications or specialized therapies may be needed.

A tailored approach works best.

Chapter Summary

Some patients require advanced or individualized treatment approaches.

Surgery may be useful in selected cases of sleep apnea.

New therapies such as nerve stimulation are becoming available.

Sleep problems in older adults require careful evaluation.

Chronic medical conditions and sleep disorders often affect each other.

Shift work and travel can disrupt normal sleep patterns.

Action Plan

- Seek specialist advice if standard treatments are not effective
- Discuss all available options with your doctor
- Review your medical conditions and medications
- Maintain consistent sleep habits whenever possible
- Plan ahead for shift work or travel
- Do not accept poor sleep as normal aging

Transition to Chapter 18

Treatment is important, but long-term success depends on maintaining good sleep over time.

In the next chapter, we will focus on how to protect your sleep and prevent problems from returning.

CHAPTER 18: Protecting Your Sleep for Life

Sleep Is Not a One-Time Fix

By now, you have understood how sleep works, what can disturb it, and how it can be treated.

The next step is just as important.

Sleep is not something you fix once and forget. It is something you maintain.

In my experience, the patients who continue to sleep well over the years are not the ones who rely on a single treatment.

They are the ones who build simple habits and follow them consistently.

Sleep improves with effort, but it stays good with consistency.

Building Habits That Last

The most powerful habit is a regular sleep schedule.

Going to bed and waking up at the same time every day keeps your internal clock stable.

Even small variations, especially on weekends, can gradually disturb this rhythm.

Daytime habits also matter.

Regular physical activity, exposure to natural light, and a structured routine support better sleep at night.

You do not need perfection. You need consistency.

Doctor's Pearl

Consistency is more important than perfection.
Small daily habits create long-term results.

Preventing the Return of Sleep Problems

Many patients improve their sleep and then slowly return to old habits.

Late nights, irregular schedules, increased screen time, and stress can quietly bring back sleep problems.

The key is early awareness.

If you notice:

- Taking longer to fall asleep
- Waking up more frequently
- Feeling tired again

take it seriously.

Returning to basic habits early can prevent the problem from becoming established again.

Staying Consistent With Treatment

For patients using treatments such as CPAP or medications, consistency is essential.

Using CPAP regularly, even when you feel better, is important.

The benefit continues only as long as the treatment continues.

Medications should be used as prescribed and reviewed regularly.

Follow-up visits allow adjustments and ensure that treatment remains effective.

Doctor's Pearl

Stopping treatment too early often brings the problem back.
Stay consistent, even when you feel better.

The Role of Family and Environment

Sleep is influenced by the environment around you.

A calm and quiet home environment supports better sleep.

Family members can help by maintaining similar routines and reducing disturbances at night.

A bed partner may also notice early signs of sleep problems, such as snoring or restlessness.

Your bedroom should support sleep.

Keep it comfortable, quiet, and free from unnecessary distractions.

Recognizing Early Warning Signs

Even with the best habits, sleep problems can return.

Watch for early signs:

- Difficulty falling asleep
- Frequent awakenings
- Daytime fatigue
- Mood changes

In patients with sleep apnea, return of snoring or sleepiness may indicate that treatment needs adjustment.

Early recognition allows early correction.

Doctor's Pearl

Small changes in sleep are early warning signals.
Do not ignore them.

Staying Motivated Over Time

Maintaining good sleep habits requires motivation.

When sleep improves, it is easy to relax and neglect these habits.

Over time, this can undo progress.

I often remind my patients to focus on how they feel when they sleep well.

Better energy, clearer thinking, and improved mood are strong motivators.

Sleep is not just about avoiding problems. It is about improving quality of life.

Chapter Summary

Good sleep requires ongoing care and consistency.

A regular sleep schedule is essential.

Early recognition of problems helps prevent relapse.

Consistent use of treatments is necessary for long-term benefit.

Family and environment play an important role.

Maintaining motivation helps sustain good sleep habits.

Action Plan

- Maintain a consistent sleep and wake schedule
- Reinforce good habits at the first sign of difficulty
- Use treatments regularly as prescribed
- Keep your sleep environment calm and comfortable
- Monitor changes in your sleep pattern
- Follow up with your doctor when needed

Transition to Chapter 19

You now understand how to maintain good sleep over time.

The next step is to bring everything together into a simple and practical plan.

In the next chapter, we will create a clear, step-by-step approach that you can start using immediately.

CHAPTER 19: A Simple, Practical Plan to Sleep Better

Turning Knowledge Into Action

By now, you understand sleep in a clear and meaningful way.

You know what healthy sleep looks like. You understand what can go wrong and how it affects the body and mind. You also know the different ways sleep problems can be treated.

The next step is very important.

You have to put this knowledge into action.

Most patients do not need complicated instructions. They need a simple, practical plan that they can follow.

I often tell my patients, "Do not try to change everything at once. Start small, stay consistent, and build gradually."

This chapter gives you that plan.

A Simple 7-Day Reset

This short plan is designed to help you begin.

It is not meant to be perfect. It is meant to get you started.

Day 1 and Day 2
Fix your wake-up time. Choose a time and follow it every day, even after a poor night's sleep.

Day 3 and Day 4
Reduce caffeine, especially in the afternoon and evening. Begin limiting screen use at least one hour before bedtime.

Day 5
Create a simple bedtime routine. Dim the lights. Avoid stimulating activities. Allow your mind to slow down.

Day 6
Review your sleep environment. Make sure your bedroom is quiet, dark, and comfortable.

Day 7
Pause and observe. Notice how you feel during the day. Even small improvements are meaningful.

Doctor's Pearl

Do not wait for the perfect plan.
Start with small changes and build from there.

A 30-Day Plan for Lasting Change

Short-term improvement is encouraging, but lasting change requires consistency.

Week 1
Focus on regular sleep and wake times. Build the basic foundation.

Week 2
Add relaxation techniques and a calming bedtime routine.

Week 3
Address specific habits such as late meals, alcohol use, irregular schedules, or excessive screen time.

Week 4
Strengthen what is working. Adjust what is not. Maintain consistency.

By the end of this period, many patients begin to notice real improvement.

Tracking Your Progress Without Stress

It is helpful to observe your sleep, but not to become overly focused on it.

A simple sleep diary is enough.

Record:

- Bedtime

- Wake-up time
- How you feel during the day

Avoid watching the clock during the night. This increases anxiety and makes sleep more difficult.

Sleep improves best in a calm, steady environment.

Handling Common Challenges

Improving sleep is not always a straight path.

Some nights will be better than others.

Frustration is common, especially when improvement is not immediate.

It is important to remember that sleep improves gradually.

Consistency is often the biggest challenge.

Weekends, travel, and social activities can disrupt your routine.

The key is to return to your routine as soon as possible.

Doctor's Pearl

A few bad nights do not mean failure.
What matters is returning to your routine.

When to Seek Help

Many people improve with these steps.

However, not everyone does.

If sleep problems continue despite consistent effort, medical evaluation is important.

Conditions such as sleep apnea, chronic insomnia, or restless legs syndrome may require specific treatment.

Seeking help early can prevent long-term problems.

Staying Motivated

Motivation becomes easier when you begin to feel the benefits.

Better energy, clearer thinking, and improved mood reinforce your efforts.

Set realistic expectations.

Focus on steady improvement, not perfection.

Sleep is not just about rest. It is about improving your daily life.

Chapter Summary

A simple, structured plan can improve sleep.

Small, consistent changes are more effective than sudden major changes.

A 7-day reset helps you begin.

A 30-day plan builds lasting habits.

Tracking sleep should be simple and not stressful.

Medical help is needed if problems persist.

Action Plan

- Fix a consistent wake-up time starting today
- Reduce caffeine and screen use in the evening
- Create a calming bedtime routine
- Keep a simple sleep diary
- Stay consistent even after a poor night
- Seek medical advice if needed

Transition to Chapter 20

You now have both the knowledge and the tools to improve your sleep.

In the final chapter, we will bring everything together and focus on the most important message of this book.

How better sleep can lead to a healthier and more fulfilling life.

CHAPTER 20: Final Thoughts – Better Sleep, Better Health, Better Life

A Simple Truth Worth Remembering

After everything we have discussed in this book, I would like to leave you with one simple and powerful truth.

Sleep is not a luxury. It is a basic human need.

In my years of medical practice, I have seen how deeply sleep affects every part of life. When sleep improves, patients begin to feel better, think more clearly, and function more efficiently. When sleep is poor, both the body and the mind begin to struggle.

Many people adjust their lives around poor sleep. They accept fatigue, reduced energy, and lack of focus as normal.

But it does not have to be this way.

With the right understanding and steady effort, sleep can improve.

Seeing Sleep as a Core Part of Health

We often speak about diet and exercise as essential pillars of health.

Sleep belongs in the same category.

Without good sleep, even the best diet and exercise plan cannot give full benefit.

Sleep supports:

- Heart health
- Brain function
- Metabolism
- Emotional balance

When patients begin to take sleep seriously, I often see improvement in many other areas of their health.

Sleep is not separate from health. It is part of it.

Doctor's Pearl

You can improve your health in many ways, but without good sleep, the results will always be limited.

The Power of Small, Consistent Changes

One of the most encouraging aspects of sleep care is that improvement does not require complexity.

Simple steps, when followed consistently, can make a meaningful difference.

A regular sleep schedule, reduced screen use in the evening, a calm bedtime routine, and attention to daily habits can gradually restore healthy sleep.

These are not dramatic changes.

They are practical, sustainable changes.

Over time, they become part of your lifestyle.

If You Have Struggled for a Long Time

Some readers may feel discouraged.

They may have had poor sleep for years.

To them, I want to say this clearly.

Improvement is possible.

I have seen many patients who struggled for a long time regain restful sleep with the right approach.

It may take time. It may require patience. But progress can be made.

Do not lose hope.

Doctor's Pearl

Even long-standing sleep problems can improve. Patience and consistency are the key.

A Doctor's Practical Advice

Let me leave you with a few simple points.

Take your sleep seriously. Do not ignore persistent problems.

Pay attention to how you feel during the day. Your daytime function reflects your nighttime sleep.

Make small changes and stay consistent. Do not expect immediate results.

Seek medical help when needed. Many sleep disorders are treatable.

And remember one important thing.

Sleep cannot be forced, but it can be supported.

When you create the right conditions, your body responds.

Your Next Step Begins Today

You do not need to wait for the right time.

Start today.

Choose one or two changes. Keep your plan simple. Stay steady.

Observe how you feel over time.

Make sleep a priority, not an afterthought.

Chapter Summary

Sleep is a fundamental part of health.

It supports physical, mental, and emotional well-being.

Simple, consistent habits can lead to meaningful improvement.

Even long-standing sleep problems can improve with the right approach.

Taking sleep seriously improves overall quality of life.

Action Plan

- Start with one simple change today
- Maintain a consistent sleep schedule
- Reduce late-night stimulation
- Monitor your daytime energy
- Seek help if sleep problems persist
- Stay committed to long-term sleep health

Closing Thought

Better sleep is not just about resting at night.

It is about living better during the day.

When you sleep well, your mind is clearer, your body is stronger, and your life feels more balanced.

Take care of your sleep, and it will take care of you.

APPENDIX 1: A 30-Day Plan to Improve Your Sleep

A Simple, Realistic Way to Begin

In my experience, patients often try to change too many things at once. That usually does not work.

Sleep improves best when changes are simple, steady, and consistent.

This 30-day plan is designed to help you build better sleep habits step by step, without feeling overwhelmed.

Week 1: Reset Your Body Clock

Start with the most important habit.

- Fix a regular wake-up time and follow it every day, including weekends
- Go to bed only when you feel sleepy
- Avoid daytime naps if you are struggling with insomnia
- Reduce caffeine after early afternoon

Your goal this week is simple.

Train your body to wake up at a consistent time.

Week 2: Improve Your Sleep Environment and Routine

Now focus on preparing your body for sleep.

- Keep your bedroom quiet, dark, and comfortably cool
- Avoid using your phone or watching TV in bed
- Start a calm routine 30 to 60 minutes before bedtime
- Reduce exposure to bright screens in the evening

This week is about sending a clear signal to your body that it is time to rest.

Week 3: Calm the Mind

At this stage, many patients notice that their biggest challenge is not the body, but the mind.

- Practice slow breathing or simple relaxation techniques
- Avoid stressful discussions or work close to bedtime
- Write down worries or next-day tasks earlier in the evening
- Continue your regular sleep schedule

The goal is to quiet the mind before sleep.

Week 4: Strengthen and Maintain

Now you begin to build long-term habits.

- Continue all the positive steps from previous weeks
- Notice what is helping and continue it
- Avoid returning to irregular sleep patterns
- Stay consistent, even on weekends

This is where improvement becomes more stable.

Doctor’s Pearl

Sleep improves gradually.
Do not look for perfection. Look for steady progress.

What You Should Expect

- Improvement may be gradual
- Some nights will still be difficult
- Consistency matters more than results on any single night

Stay patient. The body responds over time.

APPENDIX 2: A Simple Sleep Diary

Why a Sleep Diary Helps

Many patients are surprised when they begin to track their sleep.

Patterns become clearer. Small problems become easier to recognize.

A sleep diary is not complicated, and it does not take much time.

But it can be very useful.

How to Use It

Keep this diary for one to two weeks.

Each morning, write down:

- What time you went to bed
- How long it took you to fall asleep (estimate)
- How many times you woke up
- What time you woke up in the morning
- How rested you felt

Also note during the day:

- Daytime sleepiness (mild, moderate, severe)
- Any naps
- Caffeine or alcohol intake

Do not worry about exact numbers. Estimates are enough.

Simple Daily Format

Date: ___________

Time to bed: ___________
Estimated time to fall asleep: ___________
Night awakenings: ___________
Wake-up time: ___________

Morning feeling: Refreshed / Somewhat tired / Very tired

Daytime sleepiness: None / Mild / Moderate / Severe

Notes: ____________________________

Doctor's Pearl

The sleep diary is a guide, not a test.
Use it to understand your sleep, not to judge it.

APPENDIX 3: When to Seek Medical Help – A Practical Checklist

Do Not Ignore These Symptoms

You should consider medical evaluation if you notice:

- Loud or regular snoring
- Pauses in breathing during sleep
- Choking or gasping at night
- Persistent daytime sleepiness
- Difficulty staying awake during routine activities
- Trouble falling asleep or staying asleep for several weeks
- Unusual movements or behaviors during sleep
- An uncomfortable urge to move your legs at night

These are not minor symptoms. They often point to treatable conditions.

Situations That Need Early Attention

Seek medical advice sooner if you have:

- High blood pressure that is difficult to control

- Heart disease
- Diabetes
- Obesity
- A history of stroke
- Regular use of sedatives or pain medications

In these situations, sleep problems can worsen overall health.

What to Expect From Your Doctor

Your doctor will usually:

- Ask detailed questions about your sleep
- Review your medical history
- Recommend a sleep study if needed
- Suggest appropriate treatment

In some cases, you may be referred to a sleep specialist.

Doctor's Pearl

Do not wait until sleep problems become severe.
Early evaluation often leads to simple solutions.

Final Thought on Appendixes

These tools are meant to be used, not just read.

Return to them when needed.

Use them as a guide in your daily life.

Sleep improves when understanding turns into action.

Thank You and Please Review the Book

Thank you for taking the time to read this book. I sincerely hope it has helped you understand your health a little more clearly and has given you practical, everyday steps you can follow with confidence. If you found this book helpful, **I would truly appreciate it if you could leave a brief and honest review.** Even a few lines sharing your experience can make a meaningful difference. Your feedback helps other readers find reliable, trustworthy health information and supports them in making better decisions for themselves and their families.

Warm regards,

Dr Prabhat Das

Continue your Healthcare Journey with these Books

Good health is a journey, not a single step. It is not achieved in one day or with one book. That is why I created the "Better Health with Dr Das Series", with each book addressing a different common condition. If you would like easy, practical guidance on other everyday health concerns, you may wish to explore the rest of books in this series.

Books in this series:

- Better Health starts Here: A Doctor's Guide to Staying Healthy After 40
- A Doctor's Easy Guide to Understanding & Managing OBESITY
- Doctor, What DIET Is Best for Me?
- Doctor, Why Can't I Lose Weight? A Doctor's Guide to Safe & Sustainable Weight Loss)
- A Doctor's Easy Guide to GLP-1 for Obesity
- A Doctor's Easy Guide to Understanding & Managing HIGH BLOOD PRESSURE
- A Doctor's Guide to Living Well With DIABETES
- A Doctor's Guide to Understanding & Managing THYROID DISEASES
- A Doctor's Guide to Understanding & Managing HIGH CHOLESTEROL
- A Doctor's Practical Guide to HEART HEALTH After 40: How to Protect Your Heart & Live Longer
- A Doctor's Guide to Healing & Reversing FATTY LIVER DISEASE: Simple, Natural & Science-Based Steps to Reduce Liver Fat and Prevent Complications

- Control Your ACID REFLUX, HEARTBURN & GERD: A Doctor's Practical Guide that Works
- Live Comfortably with IRRITABLE BOWEL SYNDROME: A Doctor's Practical Guide to Understanding & Managing IBS
- A Doctor's Practical Guide to Understanding & Managing GALLBLADDER STONES & OTHER PROBLEMS
- Take Control of COPD: A Doctor's Practical Guide to Better Breathing
- Living Better with ASTHMA: A Doctor's Practical Guide to Asthma Control
- SLEEP APNEA, INSOMNIA & OTHER SLEEP PROBLEMS: A Doctor's Practical Guide to Better Sleep & Better Health
- KIDNEY STONES: A Doctor's Practical Guide to Prevention & Care
- Protect Your KIDNEYS: A Doctor's Practical Guide to Kidney Health & Prevention
- PROSTATE HEALTH After 40: A Doctor's Practical Guide to Early Detection & Care
- ARTHRITIS: A Doctor's Practical Guide to Pain Control & Mobility
- A Doctor's Practical Guide to Fixing BACK PAIN Step by Step
- A Doctor's Practical Guide to Understanding & Managing GOUT & URIC ACID and Preventing Complications
- HEALTHY SKIN & COMMON SKIN PROBLEMS: A Doctor's Practical Guide to Skin Care
- DEMENTIA & MEMORY LOSS: A Doctor's Practical Guide to Prevention & Management
- Doctor, Why Am I TIRED All the Time? Fixing Fatigue & Getting Your Energy Back

9 781971 672496

Printed by Libri Plureos GmbH in Hamburg,
Germany